CONTENTS

Cover Photo: Front entrance Maforki Ebola Treatment Unit with Ebola survivor supplies laid out for distribution. Foreground right is the Ebola survivor tree on which patients tied their personal survivor ribbons.

ACKNOWLEDGMENTS

The author would like to acknowledge the Sierra Leone government and especially the Port Loko district for their critical support of the Ebola response mission.

Prologue

Sierra Leone is the poorest country on the face of the planet. Dead last out of 206 countries. There is no ten-count for countries like Sierra Leone, no referee to pause the fight and let it regain its senses and shake off the punches while picking itself up off the mat. History has conspired against it, or more accurately, the world has conspired against it, especially western powers.

I wasn't alive to experience the excitement of being discovered or discovering new lands. You weren't either, so our shared ignorance is something we have to study away in the classroom. Here's what we know when we avail ourselves of a history lesson: Western Africa was found by the British and Portuguese, just sort of lying around and no one doing anything with it, or anything they considered worthwhile or worth respecting, so they took it. The Portuguese noted and named Sierra Leone, the northern most part of what was the Mali Empire at the time, meaning Lion Mountain. Explorers moved on and not until a century later was interest in West Africa rekindled.

During the 17th and 18th century, the British and Dutch had their interest piqued when they discovered what looked like a sturdy people, the sort you could teach your language, hook up to a plow and have an excellent return on investment, just as if it were draft animal breeding stock. Historically, that interest is known as the West's great shame, the slave trade. Both countries spent a better part of the 18th century ravaging West Africa's coastline, seizing human loot along the Grain, Ivory, Gold and Slave coasts, transporting it in the hulls of great commercial and martial navies to plantations and servant quarters throughout the British Empire. Captives became sugar cutters in the Caribbean, cotton and farm hands in North

America, servants, smiths, and livery labor for all manner of trades, skilled and menial, to anyone who plopped down the Crowns and Pounds anywhere in the world that mattered in the 1700's. Sierra Leone was in the thick of it.

In the early 19th century, Britain grew a conscience and outlawed slavery in Great Britain while the Dutch continued acting out. Britain didn't just refrain from turning men into property; they actually made attempts at atonement by intercepting commercial slave ships from other countries to repatriate the captives back to West Africa. Sierra Leone was one such busy hub. Freetown was established post American Revolution when thousands of slaves had acquired their freedom fighting the insurgent colonial rebels in the name of the King. The sole purpose of these repatriating efforts, led in large part by John Wesley, the British theologian responsible for the evangelical movement, motivated by issues of prison reform and abolition, was to return the newly freed back to their ancestral lands.

The first few hundred who arrived in Freetown made a go of it for about twenty seconds before succumbing to the Four Horseman. Not to be denied, there were a great many left over newly freed men milling about London and what is now Nova Scotia, not doing well. From this pool, more were lotteried out to Freetown to roll the dice. This time, there were enough men and resources to achieve a critical mass that became a city.

What is it that men do to achieve a measure of a living, a sustainable living? Most often, they fall back on what they know and understand. What was it these new settlers of Sierra Leone understood? Slavery. Soon enough, they mastered the trade. White and black freemen saw no color in one another except the color of gold. Together they conspired, capturing indigenous peoples from the Temne, Sherbro and Limba chiefdoms by ambush, chase, whip, dog, horse and chain. By the technological standards of the day, these locals were no match for the newly freed brand of slave traders, frog marched miles upon days to the coastline into the maw of timbered wind powered dungeons. When sailors above pissed the deck, it rained urine on the meat locker stalls where the cargo was salted away, washing the last of the free red soil of the captives' homeland off their diminishing shoulders.

Years passed and the slave trade diminished as countries followed Britain's lead in outlawing the practice. The last great importer of human product

3

eventually fought a violent civil war where one side fought for the right of men not to be property and the other side fought for the right of men to be property. Sierra Leoneans certainly had opinions on the matter, but mostly it was an ocean away and something of interest, only a passing one. Tropical conditions imposed more immediate concerns while the political evolution of the country under British rule rolled on.

Viruses, bacteria, protozoa and helminthes, competitive and symbiotic, fought for occupation in a tentament shouldering wave after wave of internecine warfare, famine and death. Cholera, yellow fever, malaria and tuberculosis are historical diseases in the western world but are so rare that when they occur in the 1st world, they garner headlines. In Sierra Leone these diseases are alive, well and ever present alongside what are considered the neglected diseases i.e. diseases the West has little firsthand experience with on any level, diseases that are not on the radar of governments, nongovernmental aid organizations and other charities. Thousands die annually. While 1st world medicine made great strides in disease control with simple hygiene, pollution controls, nutrition, pharmaceuticals and treatment regimens, 3rd world diseases enjoyed safety in the obscurity of being 3rd world. In no small part, this obscurity was due to lack of anything profitable worth garnering the attention of the 1st world and, when it did, minerals like gold, copper, cobalt, iron, tin or precious stones, were stripped. A lack of strong central government allowed the stripping of these resources with no due regard for the health of the local populations. Get in. Get it out. Get home. Forget. Repeat. Thus, Sierra Leone was left to fend for itself.

After obtaining independence in 1961 from the British and surviving a trifecta of coups in a 13 month period in 1967-'68, civil wars popped up several times to roll back any social gains. While the rest of the world built roads, bridges, hospitals and schools, incubated national and private business, Sierra Leone would step ahead two steps, step back two. The infrastructure is essentially corrugated tin pinned to sticks. Cinder block is the national stone, nearly as ubiquitous as the sticks used to build market stalls, homes and other personal and small commercial shelter. In this construction scene, enmeshed into a chaotic political paradigm, hospitals and clinics come and go with the arrival or disappearance of a doctor, a rare profession. Two to three doctors for every 100,000 people will do that, their presence turning whatever building they are in into a hospital, their absence turning the same building into a place where one cannot find high skilled medical care, leaving patients to wait for days or weeks to linger.

Into this vacuum comes the traditional faith healers, who have less than exciting success dealing with endemic malaria, TB, yellow fever or the arm's length litany of diseases that thrive in sub Saharan Africa. What is a patient to do under these circumstances? Pain and fear are powerful motivators, causing people to seek out every possible remedy when the tried and true are absent. There is no blame to put on these individuals. If anything, there should be admiration that they are willing to risk various concoctions and treatments by fire, cutting and breaking.

This competition with 1st world medicine flourishes precisely due to the lack of 1st world medicine and the education and knowledge distributed with its presence. Female genital mutilation, a long practiced tradition of circumcising the clitoris of pubescent girls, approaches 90% by some estimates in Sierra Leone. Traditional midwives or healers fail to employ clean technique, let alone sterile technique, and may use the kitchen knife or sharp piece of metal, absent that, a piece of sharp broken glass or other object, for the surgery. No anesthetic is used and infections too often set in, sometimes killing the patient. It is a brutal tradition that 1st world trained doctors in Sierra Leone counsel heavily against on several grounds, not the least of which is medical along with the philosophical regards individual autonomy. However, the doctors are not present. Disease and ignorance has the upper hand. Tradition is the respected knowledge simply because it is available. Newer ideas are more a curiosity than a mainstream thinking. It is into this scene, this theater, forest and jungles about the villages, diseases unknown appear and disappear, not understood when they arrive and, too often, just as unknown when they disappear.

Diseases like HIV, now pandemic, came out of the jungles of Africa where the daily bread is still often bush meat, meaning monkeys and bats. Ebola, appearing in December 2013 in West Africa, traveled into Sierra Leone. With its crushing poverty, traditional burial practices, lack of medical infrastructure and weak political controls, Sierra Leone was primed for a hit in the viral lottery.

What It Is, Is It Makes You Bleed

Ebola is actually a class of viruses similar to the Marburg virus, a hemorrhagic virus, meaning the victim essentially drowns in their own fluids and/or bleeds to death internally. Some media reports concocted imagery of massive external bleeding when in fact there is very little visible bleeding, even in the most dire cases.

The first known case popped up in 1976 in Zaire (Democratic Republic of Congo) and several others appeared shortly after in Sudan. As quickly as it appeared, it melted away. In 1994, necropsies performed on chimpanzees found dead in the Tai Forest of Ivory Coast, all signs pointed to the same disease which appeared in 1976 in Zaire and Sudan. The chimpanzees examined are known to consume the meat of other monkeys, namely the western red monkey. At least one worker performing necropsies was infected who later went on to recover fully. In 1989, in Reston, Virginia, an Ebola type outbreak occurred amongst primates housed at a research laboratory; these primates were imported from the Philippines. Later, it was found that other primates at several facilities in the US, along with one in Italy, also acquired primates from the same Philippine supplier that were found to be infected. The literature on this particular outbreak seems to take pains that it is sufficiently different from the other four known types of Ebola viruses, but there are enough similarities that it should merit mention.

Since 1994, several other outbreaks in Africa were observed in chimpanzee and gorilla populations. Researchers scoured the jungles and began testing various animals and plants to see if they could get a handle on the Ebola virus reservoir, the animal that could house the virus without succumbing yet unleash its deadliness should the animal be contacted in some manner, such as eating it. What they came up with is that the most likely candidates are three species of fruit bats. While meat is generally a very small part of monkey diets, they have been seen eating the meat of other monkeys and small mammals. Fruit bats seemingly are able to carry the Ebola virus without consequence. However, when a primate mammal, such as a monkey or human, consumes an infected fruit bat, they are in danger of experiencing the Ebola virus' full consequences.

In 2007, the Ebola virus popped up again in humans in Uganda, several hundred people were infected and about 150 succumbed. Like before, as mysteriously as it appeared, it melted away and out of the human population.   In the meantime, researchers were studying every possible mode of transmission and possible reservoir, be it plant, animal or inanimate. Researchers hacked thru mosquito infested jungle, stuck their heads in pitch black caves filled with animal waste, tramped shorelines of rivers, lakes, bays and oceans dodging crocodiles, all the time enveloped in a perpetual sweat of tropical humidity and their own. What they found was, by all accounts, it did not appear to be a very intelligent virus; it had the suicidal tendency to kill off the infected target, a poor way to propagate by any definition. Based on this tendency, some researchers call it a 'stupid' virus, and the fact that it is an RNA virus with about only 27 discernible genetic parts. Viruses such as the rhinovirus, i.e. common cold, are DNA viruses with thousands of identifiable genetic parts.

In the world of the virus, not only does Ebola lack smarts, it lacks ambition. In other words, it's hard to catch because it is not airborne, needs very specific conditions to survive such as the right temperature and a nice, fresh supply of cells to infect and breed.   Deceased animals cool off and cells like macrophages and leukocytes, a primary target of Ebola, stop coming because where they lived and bred is now dead and so the virus dies, too. On the upside for the virus, the victim being dead gives it about 3 to 4 days where it can still use a person's cellular infrastructure to reproduce. West Africa is basically equatorial,   running in the 80's and 90's temperature range, so conditions keep a deceased victim warm enough for the virus to call home.

With what we know from above, the Ebola virus is likely transmitted into the human population by eating freshly deceased fruit bats or primates in what is commonly referred to as bush meat. What sounds repulsive to you or me is another man's required nutrition, and that nutrition is in the bounty of the forest for the taking. While monkey meat or fruit bat is often thrown into a stew and cooked at temperatures that would normally kill the Ebola virus, someone first needs to hunt that bat or chimp, kill it with a trauma such as an arrow, gun slug or club, then skin it up with a knife. The animal reservoir for the Ebola virus is dead but the conditions for the virus are not, meaning that as the raw meat and blood are prepared, they are potentially infectious.

I cannot speak to the nuances of bush meat culinary technique, nor preferred manner of serving, but if it is at all like western meat variability of preference, meaning some of us like our steaks red and bloody while others

7

want it nearly charcoaled. I'd venture to posit that some bush meat stews had meat cool enough not to kill off the virus, that some consumers of the meat enjoyed it el dente, such as where I grew up in northern Wisconsin, where on Christmas Eve afternoons the local taverns would serve wildcat, sandwiches of onions and raw hamburger smothered in salt and pepper.

It is under this scenario in December 2013, a 2-year-old boy in the remote Guinean village of Meliandou fell ill with a mysterious illness characterized by fever, black stools, and vomiting. Two days later, he was dead. Then more were dead. No one knew what was happening as the sick were misdiagnosed as being malaria or cholera infected. In fact, some blood samples from patients very specifically tested for cholera. As quickly as it popped up, the outbreaks faded away.

The peoples of Guinea, Liberia and Sierra Leone freely cross the border near the village of Meliandou. For three months, the missed diagnosis gave free reign for conditions to continue for the Zaire Ebola virus to spread. Governments and doctors, used to dealing with cholera and malaria, both which strongly mimic Ebola, were not at all suspicious that what was happening was something other than the usual deadly infectious diseases that dominated the region. In March, 2014, Doctors Without Borders physicians, in conjunction with World Health Organization physicians who were in the area to deal with a particularly bad malaria outbreak, sent off samples to Geneva for more in depth investigation and the Zaire strain of Ebola virus was confirmed. However, what use is sounding the fire bell if all you have is a bucket brigade. MSF (Medicine sans Frontiers aka Doctors Without Borders) was ill equipped for this type of outbreak and, frustratingly, the governments of Liberia, Sierra Leone and Guinea were even less equipped. Soon it would become a numbers game. In Vegas parlance, those numbers made Ebola a dead ringer bet to win the race, especially since it was out of the barn door, and no one knew for three months that anything escaped the barn, or that they even had something in the barn that could escape. Eventually, world media noticed the story and soon a curiosity of West Africa became a worldwide concern. That's where I and the people I worked with and come into this story.

It's All Over the News

My awareness of the outbreak happened around June, 2014. I had heard of Liberia and knew it was in West Africa, though I certainly could not say that about Sierra Leone or Guinea. The languages of Temne and Krio, spoken widely in West Africa, were new to me, nor was I at all aware of its history outside knowing, vaguely, concerned United States citizens established Liberia as a home for the repatriation of freed American slaves. This began in the early 1800's, so that freed slaves, by their presence, would not excite the enslaved population, enabling slave owners. The same repatriation efforts resulting from manumission was a Quaker objective, in line with their abolitionist and liberal beliefs of human rights. For me, worrying about Ebola an ocean and two degrees of economic development away wasn't even a passing interest.

The news stories filtered out over the summer and were part of a media diet for a large part of the world. However, no one in political circles was overly concerned since the countries of West Africa are not large trading partners or a hot tourist destination. There is something peculiarly American about disaster stories. Maybe our lives are generally so stable in the developed world, we've become bored and crave the visceral excitement and drama of the plight of others. Naturally, American media, masters of hyperbole toward the sensational, worked this new ground in an attempt to sate viewer's entertainment fix.

Internet comment boards heated up in late August, 2014 as the Ebola infection rates climbed. Many of the comments expressed a sense of doom where, in toto, the comments sections were more venues for mass hysteria than insights on current events. Respectable journalistic outlets, like the Washington Post or New York Times, went into detail how Ebola spread, the very low odds of it taking hold in Europe or North America. Readers were dismissive and hostile, claiming the media was carrying water as part of a government conspiracy to hide the true nature and spread of the disease. Certain media outlets, though, per the black helicopter crowd, were very trusted, namely the entertainment niche of political talk radio and cable news. The Beck's and Rush's were more than game to feed their listeners with 'facts' that were often nothing more than half-truths at best. One of the most popular was that the US government and Obama Administration were deliberately encouraging illegal immigrant children to cross the US-Mexican border, then forbidding health screenings of these children, thus deliberately creating a situation where Ebola could sneak in and take hold. Millions bought into this nonsense.

A game I would play was to listen to talk radio and its lineup of blowhards, seeing how long it would take for them posit a wild speculation as fact regards the Ebola developments. Usually, it took about a minute before they would say something entirely wrong, such as Ebola is an airborne disease or that terrorists were possibly sending infected Ebola patients across the borders. If stupidity, ignorance and irrational fear are diseases, then such entertainment commentary, posing as journalism, is a vector and every building owned by muckrakers is one huge nosocomial infection.

Soon, politicians were stumbling over one another to capitalize on unwarranted fear, demanding all Ebola infected nations quarantined with no one in or out, regardless of actual health status. There were calls that if someone was from West Africa, they were to be immediately put into a 21 day quarantine or deported back to country of origin, a tough task when no one was supposed to be allowed in or out. When reason dies it is likely not for a rational reason.

Soon, New Jersey Governor Chris Christie had a live one on his hands, a nurse who spent several weeks in West Africa working with Ebola cases who came home via Newark Liberty International Airport. Kaci Hickox was stopped and seized after answering questions about from where she traveled, and what she was doing in the country of her port of egress, truthfully revealing she was in West Africa's Sierra Leone, and had close and/or direct contact with Ebola patients. Never mind she was meticulous about infection control while in Sierra Leone attending to victims of the disease, or that she was afebrile, negative for coughing, hiccupping, red eyes, unexplained nausea, vomiting or diarrhea, New Jersey decided to treat her as if she was actually diagnosed with full blown Ebola, imprisoning her in a tent in a hospital parking lot. Eventually, enough medical professionals were heard over the din to force a more rational approach and Kaci Hickox was relieved of her quarantine in New Jersey, allowed to return home to Maine. Another mini drama ensued when Ms. Hickox decided to go for a country bike ride on a late fall Maine day with her partner. Being America, this ended up in court where the judge found the quarantine rules overly onerous and based more on political expediency than actual medical

gold embossed bluebook, split to the inside pages, and it is spelled out with official font of the The United States of America, 'This is who I am.'

The Sierra Leone visa stamp was buried several pages in, reds and blues depicting the national seal, filled in with various dates of when I was welcome and when I was expected to go home.

Our time passed and soon we were shuttled through town to the airport, the first step of several concluded. At the airline check in counter, apprehension was up since the American airway system was now a case study in how to abuse customers for profit. My bag came in at exactly 49.5 lbs, a half pound under the domestic weight limit, was judged appropriately sturdy by the scanning eye of the uniformed clerk behind the desk, her hair disheveled as she puffed a blond strand out of her eyes as she copied down all my flight and travel document information into her computer.

The three docs sailed through in another line and the psych nurse was up next. The display on the scale lit up at 67 lbs for one bag and 69 lbs for the second, a stern disapproval followed, "You must be at 50 lbs. Remove what you don't want and then come back." Sandy shuffled back to a spot clear of travelers and I followed, feeling an obligation to help her get it right and make it easier for us as a group. When she opened her bag, I spotted the books. 'Bingo!' I thought. 'This will be easy enough.' But as we disengorged the bags, I saw that this was not going to be so simple. Having to toss several tens of pounds of items meant we would be leaving a fair amount of value behind.

"Books", I intoned. "Only need one or two. Pick your favorites."

"I need all of them!" she objected.

"Right now, Sandy, this is where you distinguish between want and need. Books. Gone."

She delivered and made fast work of letting go about a dozen. Next, it was on to the clothes, shoes and anything easily replaceable. Out a pair of jeans went. Empty notebooks followed. Who uses this much shampoo? Six packs of soda are dead weight and failed the cut. Rubber boots? The organization will provide those in country. Time for recheck. 12 pounds overweight between the bags.

"This is fixable." It was simple numbers for me. "Anyone else have weight issues?"

"Me," Gwyn piped up. "8 pounds. Everything here has to go with since most of it is supplies for my clinics in Sierra Leone."

"I have an extra bag and I'm still allowed one more," I tell her. "If you and Sandy can pack your things into it, I'll check it in with my baggage." Items flew in handful lumps into the bag, plumping it out and giving it heft. 37 lbs. The check in clerk deftly moved her fingers around the tag string and luggage handle, and then gave the computer one more item to memorize. Problem solved.

In the meantime, Adam was taking longer than usual to complete his check in. The clerk was going back and forth thru the side door, returning to get on the phone, then talking several desks down the line to colleagues and coming back. Adam, too, was on his phone and his easy smile was missing. This trip was like fishing: always some snags.

The Major stepped forward. Now both were on the phone. Keeping my distance to keep it simple, I tried to interpret the various frowns, huh-huhs and OK's. Neither gave any sign of resolution when they closed their phones. Now I was too curious.

"What's the hold-up?" I asked.

"I have the wrong visa. My flight is for Freetown but my visa is for Liberia." The disappointment in Adam's voice was contained but visible enough. The Major was equally subdued.

"So, now what?" I asked.

"Back to the hotel and I'll follow on another flight when they get it straightened out," Adam responded, trying to be philosophical about it all. I was learning this is the sort of bravery and rolling with the punches that international travel requires. It is in such moments you want magical powers to wish away obstacles and resolve all the mix-ups. Sadly, none of us had magical powers and Adam was going to have solve his problem the regular way of mortals with patience, meaning he would have to wait while others untangled the red tape that fashioned a noose around his trip's neck. Not even on the plane and already we lost a good man.

Adam was fast becoming the man I could commiserate with, bounce off questions and ideas, exchange information to ferret out its weaknesses and strengths. The slightly hyperbolic chatter of our small talk vanished. Gwyn and Sandy offered words of silver lining into the cloud that passed over. Drs. Galleo and Peterson already checked thru and were likely near the departing gate, unaware we had just lost a fellow traveler. The Major offered his assurances and spoke accurately for all of us that soon enough we'd see each other. I just felt terrible for Adam. Now, for a minute, I felt adrift. Forging ahead, the wound to our group cocoon healed and I felt we pulled in just a little closer to one another.

Bags checked. Documents approved. On to the plane. We all jostled and bumped our way through the other passengers and found our seats. The magic of flying that was present in my younger life of 30 years ago, was gone. All the changes in the airline industry over the past decades, the assault on airline worker wages, consolidations and poor management decisions, were now giving airline customers literally a kick in the seat of pants. Seats are smaller by a couple of inches with leg room less the same amount of inches, giving quantifiable meaning to the phrase 'less is more' in the bottom lines of airlines. 'You get less, we get more' should be the industry motto and, for all I knew, it was carved into the tabletops of every piece of furniture in all the boardrooms. The height of this thinking was the culmination of the nearly entire industry rushing to charge for bags, a cynical ploy in the world of travel that pretends travelers and luggage are exclusive of one another, that the latter is a want more than a need. It's as if changes of clothes and bathroom items are no different from a set of skies or a duffel bag full of bowling pins.

Of course, it would be too much to ask the airlines to be on time. I obsessively watch the weather during the winter months to decipher what delays might happen. Obviously, no one wants an aspiring Lindberg or Yeager to challenge an ice storm, so keeping that big hunk of aluminum on the tarmac is the only real choice. We all accept that. However, the entire country was without any notable weather events, thus being late seemed more like a test of one's will. Maybe there are secret award miles given for every hour a plane is late; I'm just the last flier in the world to know this.

Eventually, our paying mass of humanity, neatly strapped in and tucked away in our seats, is treated to the set of g forces we paid several thousand dollars for, then we are deposited into one city for a layover of several hours, soon enough into the transatlantic portion of the flight. Looking down over the Atlantic I look for ships, hoping to see a tub of steel and wonder about the men on it, wondering if the romance of the sea holds them to their jobs. Is avoiding icebergs today as important as it was in the Titanic's day? I'm sure hitting an iceberg isn't any more OK today than it was in 1912, so some poor sap is on night shift, watching out off the bow or, more likely, staring at a green screen of radar dots, making sure his dot doesn't run into some other dot. Do they, the sailors, look up at the planes and imagine where we are going? Night comes quickly flying opposite earth's rotation. A couple of movies and few chapters later into my Armstrong biography, we touchdown in Brussels, 3 hours late.

No one is smiling. Everyone has on a flyer's game face as we struggle onto a bus to take us to the connecting terminal thru the Belgian drizzle. Off in the distance, I see the neat rows of houses and the typically clean and ordered European style of living, but only a peek before we are puked up into a place called Terminal T, an expanse of nothing where you can't even get a bottle of water or a snack to nibble away your boredom and tension. Then back onto a plane.

This plane is cleaner, more pleasant somehow. Then I notice we are on the national airline of Belgium, Brussels Airlines, with the flight attendants impeccably dressed in navy blues, dress grays complimented by broaches and red kerchiefs. When I see so many beautiful people in one place, performing the same work, it comes to me that some jobs are more about projecting an image. The competence is expected but is not the product. No obvious disabilities to sympathize over with nothing remotely unattractive about any of them. If most of us were to take one these attendants home to meet our moms, the certain question would probably be, 'What does she see in you?'

I grind away in my seat, shifting here, shifting there. Relief is achieved by getting out into the aisle and taking several walks, noticing the other passengers are sleeping or trying to sleep. One or two are staring at the in-seat movie screens or trying to do computer work, maybe both at the same time. Daylight arrives and our plane continues until, finally, there is a break when the captain informs of us a landing in Conakry, Guinea.

We disembark for 45 minutes for the plane to be cleaned, and then back on for several more landings and take offs along the West Africa coast. At this point, nearly 30 hours later, you just want it to stop flying, period. Finally, there is the last stop.

It's dark outside. The plane stops on the tarmac, no terminal gateway to tie into the side of the plane, so we come off on a stairway. The air is warm and humid but is just another minor discomfort since it is not refreshing like a cool breeze would be at this point. Each person in our group turns on their human GPS to find one another out of the several hundred. I notice the groups; each has its own identifiable purpose for this trip, such as the young men with close cut hair being British soldiers coming in for the Ebola fight. Then there are the well dressed women and men who most likely are government officials, or business people that have connections within the country for many sorts of reasons, the least of not which is most certainly that this is home, Freetown, Sierra Leone. My group looks like a bunch of lost white people who landed on Mars. That would make us the aliens. I touch my head nervously as if I might accidentally find a new set of antennae sprouting and am relieved to note none.

I grab my luggage off the carousel and heft it away out of the jostling of people who are equally tired and anxious to get through customs. I recall the instruction to give no bribes, to politely inform the requestor of such that I have no authorization to do so, hoping that if it happens, I don't lay an egg and spend the night by a luggage carousel, nestling down onto the floor trying to hatch that egg.

The lines move forward quickly. The customs officials look equally tired, and just as likely would like to get it all over themselves. As ordered, I present my documents and lay them out on the shelf of the booth the official is bunkered in. He indicates passport, yellow card and visa are all neat and in order, pushing back all three to me. Eventually, he speaks, asking me to put my palm down on a screen for a scan and to stand still in front of a camera. He rebukes me not to flinch. I don't. Finally, I hear the words that all is good, "Welcome to Sierra Leone." His smile is genuine and after 30 hours in the air, it's a nice prompt that spreads a smile over my face as well.

Our group now is lugging what will be our lives for the next six weeks through and down the gangways. Two men run up to us waving stacks of bills. Do they want money from us? Antonino and Kati, who jumped onto our flight with our group of minus one, quickly round us up a little tighter. Antonino, in his completely unflustered tone and manner, instructs us this is the currency exchange. I spot out a hundred dollar bill, fresh and crisp, and in return, one of the men hands me a stack of bills that would choke a small pony. 'Wow! I'm stinkin' rich!', I think. All of us have done likewise, our comments on the bills ranging from their beauty to the quantity. Everyone wondered aloud exactly how much 10,000 Leones was worth, the denomination of each bill in each stack of 500,000 per $100US. Quick math deciphers that each 10k note is about 2 bucks, or two cans of Coke, a measure I end up stuck with for the remainder of the trip when making a purchase, counting in my head how many Cokes I was paying for whatever item it was I was considering purchasing.

Out the doors of the airport, the concrete is brief before giving way to red clay and gravel splattered with mud puddles and mud ponds for us to avoid as we catch up to our shuttle bus. Out of the crowd, a young blond woman appears and grabs us up. "No, here. Welcome everyone. Get in the van." Two commands and a greeting with no waste on the small talk. Mary is now in charge of us to see to it that her new charges, us, are put into our hotel and made ready for the car trip up to Port Loko.

The trip to the hotel in the company van is dark, but one can see enough that the market surrounding the airport is sticks and corrugated tin with a healthy population of goats and dogs who, by their looks, all share the same parents. Only men are out at this hour and they all are young, no more than 25 or so, I guess.

Finally, we pull into the hotel and are assigned rooms for the night. Things are broken, cracked, but you sense the effort of the staff to overcome the material failings through the pleasantness and almost fanatical efforts to please us. When I'm given my room key, the desk clerk gives me serious counsel, "If you find anything at all not satisfying with your room, find me, Ali, and let me know. Understand?"

"Uhm, sure, yes. I'll do that," I say, trying to put him at ease.

"So what will you do if you find something not to your liking?" Ali quizzes me.

"Find you?" I said, as if I might flunk if I gave an unsatisfactory answer.

"No! You will find me, Ali." He wasn't satisfied, continuing, "Who will you ask for?"

I wasn't going to fail this time. "I ask for you, Ali."

He breaks into a smile, all perfect teeth, and hands me my key, pointing, "111 down the hall and always ask for Ali."

I start away, lugging my bag like a tired man when I hear, "Do you need help with your bag? If you do, you know who to ask for."

"Yeah, I just ask for Ali."

With that Ali comes around the counter and before I know it he is two steps ahead of me, leading down the hall to my room, gestures at my hand for the key, unlocks the door and deposits the bag around the inside corner. Then he waits.

I get it. "Thank you, Ali," I say, peeling off a 10k note from my bankroll. He's happy and disappears down the hall back to his desk.

Finally alone to my own thoughts, I see sign one that I'm really somewhere else on the planet other than in the middle of a corn field. The mosquito net hangs over my bed, tented up with the white mesh flowing over the sides. I put down the bag to wander out to the lobby, noticing the bar. The chatter is mostly accented English with some French and German. Watching and listening is enough excitement for me, I order up a bottle of water after waiting for a few minutes, studiously ignored by the bartender, a young woman who doesn't seem particularly happy with her job since she serves me a bottle wordlessly, seemingly expecting me to read her mind on what I owe. The price of six Cokes as I keep laying down one 10k note after the other. Soon, 30k is on the bar. I just learned that drinks are U.S. priced. No 3rd world discount.

Behind me, I hear a Midwestern accent directed at me, asking, "You. Are you part of a medical team just in?" The thirtyish age woman is looking me over.

I nod, answering, "I came in with a small group from the US. We're heading up to Port Loko tomorrow morning." Then I quickly add my introduction, "By the way I'm Rick. And you are…?"

She tells me her name, and in two seconds, I forget it. A young British officer who was working the lady now appears a little worried and anxious, but he introduces himself with a firm, polite handshake as we exchange names and some quick small talk on our assignments. The woman jumps in, "I heard you in the lobby tell someone you're from the Midwest. What state?"

When I finish giving the place name, she laughs and tells me she's doing CDC contract work in the capital city just an hour south of my own home. I tell her it's OK, that the sting of living there isn't bad since I'm near a major university but I could do without the seas and seas of corn that stretch beyond the beyond. Then she switches gears completely.

"You need to be careful. Not here; this place is safe. You need to be careful when you get back home," obviously serious.

"Why's that?"

"When I was back, working down near the capital for the CDC, I was called out of work to the governor's office, supposedly to give advice on how to handle returning travelers from West Africa. When I got there, it was the governor with the Attorney General and some other dweeb with no neck. They didn't give a damn what I had to say about quarantine guidelines."

Her lips were tight and thin with no trace of a smile. I prodded her for more, "What else did they want?"

She spit out, "They *demanded*…They didn't *want* anything."

"Demanded?" I questioned, cutting her off.

"Oh, yes. Demanded. They demanded that I release any names of those I know working in West Africa with the CDC or any other US governmental or NGO. We get all of your names because we have to forward them to port authorities for when you return to the states. But that's a federal issue and not a state issue, so I told him and his sidekick that I work for the federal government and that I owe him nothing, that all the names I have are confidential. He didn't like that answer and told me they have other ways of finding out which, if true, was pretty odd since he was asking me for a list." She spit out these words with no small amount of contempt, adding, "God, our state is so damned backwards. The AG tried intimidating me by saying he could bring me into court," rolling her eyes for effect. "What a couple of knuckle draggers."

"Well," I commiserated, "politicians like that are blind to any contradictions between their rhetoric and actions. Civil liberties and individual rights are pretty far down the list judging by their actions. What you described is exactly what I expect of the uninformed and superstitious. Problem is this: Even when they are informed and disabused of bad information, they simply pretend it doesn't exist. It's like talking to a brick."

She smiled again and fiddled her drink, "Don't let those bastards get you down. If they try to give you any crap when you get home, tell 'em to stuff it."

She wasn't pulling her punches on what she thought. The Brit officer was back in the conversation and working the bartender for another round but she was ignoring him, and everyone else at the bar, before he finally tired of waiting and got off his stool, went behind the bar and opened up the cooler to serve himself. He then pulled the Merlot and poured the woman a freshener. "Sometimes you just have to take action," he grinned, raising his beer, "Cheers, mates." The bartender was buried in her phone, so even if she noticed, I don't think she really cared. We all left money on the bar to be even with the house.

Off to bed. This is not the night to stay out all hours. Anyways, I had to get a decent shower and get my Malerone onto the evening schedule now that I was in-country. Cleaned up and medicated, I headed to bed and struggled with the mosquito net to make sure no arm or leg was sticking out before relaxing, which when achieved, I found I missed having a furry, purring cat kneading my arm until sleep prevailed.
■■

Port Loko

A warm morning with a green landscape in early December is a blessing for anyone from the northern climes of the US, especially those of us who endure what are basically 6 months of cold car starts, scraping icy windshields and shoveling snowdrifts. It doesn't matter where it is at as long as it's not snow.

Everyone was fed and at the ready with their luggage. Soon enough, two Chrysler minivans were beneath the hotel entrance atrium with the drivers tossing our luggage and our greeter-guide, Mary, directing us to take seats. I noticed that the dealer stickers on the lift gate of the vans showed that the vehicles came from a dealership in Ohio, making me wonder how they managed to get it into Sierra Leone, who would go through the trouble or expense of doing so when vehicles likely could be more easily obtained from nearby countries.

Off we went thru Lungi, onto the one paved road to Port Loko. The road itself was in excellent condition, appearing not to be to more than a couple of years old, but it lacked common safety features of fog and lane lines. The countryside was still lush from the rainy season that ceased just two or three days earlier, with goats seemingly everywhere even when not near any sort of settlement. The typical expectation expats like me had of seeing thatched huts was met as there were more than a few but, by far, the dominant building material was simple arm sized sticks and logs tacked with corrugated tin. The more well off homes were constructed of cinder block, or a type of red mud brick made from the earth.

Our driver, a tall, noble-looking man of 27, a possible heir to the title of chief in his clan, was, by all accounts, happy with his job as he chatted us up. I asked his name, to which he smiled, pronouncing, "Ibrahim."

My ear didn't quite catch the annunciation, forcing me to ask again. "E-Bra-Heem," he slowly articulated, then laughed, "Like Abraham Lincoln. You know your Abraham Lincoln, correct?"

"Yeah. The question is: how do you know about Abraham Lincoln," I asked.

"We learn about all your presidents in our schools. Everyone knows who Abraham Lincoln is: even the little children know about the great Abraham Lincoln, and I am named just like him." He was obviously honored to share such a highly similar pronunciation with arguably our greatest US president. He went on, "Have you ever met President Obama? I think Obama is a great man. All of Sierra Leone loves him. Very great man."

The Major, Galleo, Gwyn and Mary found this amusing, prompting the Major to tell us how his former military assignment included greeting both presidents Bush and Obama as they exited an elevator into a secure area where their semi-annual physicals and other medical appointments were handled.

Ibrahim, practically shouting, looked back in his mirror, "So you have met Obama! I am giving a ride to a man who has met President Obama!" Ibrahim followed with questions about if he was nice or if the Major had ever his met his wife, which the Major politely answered in the positive and the negative.

"Wow. I have a man in my car who met Obama," Ibrahim bubbled. "This is a good day."

We continued with other small talk, trying to get Ibrahim to help us identify birds, asking about other wildlife such as lions, monkeys and hippos. We learned that lions were mostly gone, monkeys lived in the dense brush and avoided people, and that a man should never get in between a hippo and water or else the hippo would become alarmed and run you over. This wasn't going to be a problem since the hippos were more than a day's drive over rough roads, up near the Guinea border. Other than the minister bird, a crow like bird, black with a white V collar coming off its back and over the breast, we saw no other birds.

Other vehicles on the road were trucks hauling commercial goods, mostly what looked like bundles of palm leaves used for furniture, or an occasional fuel truck. No utility poles with electrical or phone were present, which was good for the drivers who went off the road. Judging by the number of flipped over cars off to the sides, some burned out and left to lie, it was a good thing they didn't have an immovable object to wrap their car or truck around. The number one cause of foreigner deaths in Sierra Leone, and most other African nations, is the auto wreck, due in no small part to the complete lack of formal driver training and regulated, well marked roads. The rules of the road apparently amounted to some sort of unspoken understanding of who had right of way, or what the speed limits were in any given stretch. I had yet to see a stop sign on our trip. During my entire time in country, I spotted only one, and it was because I was on a British military post near the hospital we would be working.

Ibrahim was a good driver, appropriate in speed and temperament. After an hour, we were on the outskirts of Port Loko, a community of 150,000 souls located on the Bankasoka River that flowed down into the Sierra Leone River to form the Port Loko Creek tidal basin near Freetown and Lungi. With daylight and slower driving, we meandered thru town, the lack of general public infrastructure notable and, for what there was, it was discouraging. As we crossed a bridge over the Bankasoka, visible was the incomplete concrete remains of what appeared to be an unfinished hydroelectric project that was likely big on aspirations to provide reliable power, but was stopped due to the Ebola outbreak. Would it ever be finished was a guess either way, no matter who you spoke with about the project.* For all I knew, maybe there was a very strong lobby for electricity generator dealers and manufacturers who abhorred the prospect of public utility.

*(As of September 2015 the project resumed and is 80% complete).

Dodging the ubiquitous motorcycles and pedestrians on the roads carrying loads of firewood or produce, beeping his horn so much that it would make a New York city cabbie blush, Ibrahim got us through the city center traffic circle that was the market hub for the city. Hundreds of stick and tin shacks selling fruits, fried dough, goat, fish or chicken meats, clothing, shoes, odds and ends of hardware and cell phones. Looking about, it seemed like every third business in the market had something to sell related to cell phones, be it the phones and data plans, or space on an outlet connected to a private generator to charge your phone, a thriving business for a country where hydroelectric wasn't happening.

Ibrahim pulled our van onto a potholed, damp red gravel road and passed what was one of the largest species of trees I had ever seen outside of California redwoods and Douglas fir back on the Pacific coast. You could see it covered with thumb sized thorns, provided tremendous shade, thrived in poor soil conditions and had a diameter of 10 feet at hip height. I learned this species of tree, the Kapok tree, was a local attraction in Freetown where freed slaves from Nova Scotia in the 1790's supposedly held a ceremony of thanks under such tree, now known as the Cotton tree. Later, I found out online that the Kapok is also found in Mexico, South America and the Caribbean. Just as I could no longer spy the tree out my window, we were at a formidable iron gate and Ibrahim was stomping on the horn.

The gate opened into a courtyard with an outdoor patio and hand pump well. The walls of the compound were studded with broken glass and barbed wire, giving 'home' a not so welcoming feeling. Before we could exit the car, several young men encircled the car and opened our doors, grabbed our bags and started running them into the lobby. Mary was out and on her phone, reminding us we would be given rooms followed by going to the government hospital to meet up with Dr. Thiede, Antonino and Kati for some quick training and tours.

My room was nice enough with a queen size bed, tiled floors and small bathroom that was bathroom more in name than function. A quick check of the plumbing unmasked a sink with no running water and toilet that didn't flush. In all, there were maybe 20 rooms in what appeared to be an old hotel that was mothballed until the organization found it and rented it for our comfort. We could get cozy in here, I thought.

All the young men introduced themselves with names I could not quite grasp with my Midwestern ear, followed by the typical back and forth between us all repeating our names slowly until we did comprehend. Then back into the van, just as quickly as we arrived it seemed, Ibrahim backtracked us down to the government hospital we had passed earlier. Again, the obligatory horn stomping came on and the gates opened to let us through. By far, the hospital was the nicest building I had seen with fresh white walls, porches and veranda, topped with stylish royal blue steel roofing that would be the envy of your neighbors back in the States. Mary ushered us inside where we were greeted by a grizzly looking fellow who was a real doctor, an Ob-Gyn fellow.

Much more soft spoken than his sun weathered, unshaven, tattered work street clothes would lead a person to believe, David made quick introductions and stated our purpose: we would be practicing donning and doffing and, in the meantime, have lunch until the other half of our cohorts arrived.

In the middle of our ham and egg burritos specially ordered 3 hours before our arrival, a lag time that was common and getting longer due to the alleged perfectionism of the local chef who prepared the fare, Sandy and David showed up. We were good to go.

We opened the boxes of Tyvek biohazard suits, grabbing one as instructed. Dr. Thiede asked for three of us to step forward to be the first to go through the donning and doffing process. One could sense that we were all feeling out our positions with one another. At this point, no one wanted to appear to be the eager beaver know it all or a wallflower that needed to be peeled out of the corner to do something. Three of us volunteered to be the ones who made the glaring errors that could get a health person killed.

Dr. Thiede talked us through the donning, instructing us how to shoelessly don the body suit, zip to the top, peel off the zipper seal tape and tamp shut. Next, was rubber boots on with suit legs covering the boot rise. Now the hair net. Easy enough. Now fingers through the finger tabs to keep the sleeves down followed by the N-95 mask and hood up. Finally two sets of surgical gloves and the visor. Ready to go? No, we needed to inspect each other for errors or tears, anywhere possible virus could settle on us through a breech. Now we were ready.

"OK, that's the easy part," David near whispered. "I want you to stay like that for 20 minutes or so while I go and take care of a couple of phone calls. I promise to be right back." His smile foreshadowed enough.

The first immediate difficulty was the mask inhibiting our speech, causing the other party to have to strain to decipher our words. Even though we were in a room with an actual ceiling fan, a sort of rarity in

Sierra Leone, the beads and creeks of sweat started to moisten our clothes. Several minutes later, our masks began to fill with moisture and an audible rattle if you breathed hard enough. For anyone who was claustrophobic this would be a nightmare.

David wandered back from outside. "Warm enough yet or would you like to spend some more time inside your plastic bags?" No one agreed to more.

"Smart," David nodded. "Now comes the money portion of all this. Doffing is predictable and by the book. You will learn this and you will memorize it. If you were inside, a sprayer would have been following and spraying you with what concentration of bleach?"

In unison, the room chanted, "Zero point five percent."

"Well, good. We all know that," David agreed. "Now, you are at the doffing station and the first thing you'll do is to do exactly as the sprayer tells you. He will you ask to spread eagle, then turn and put your hands out for you to wash. Then he'll spray your boots, each sole up as he instructs..." He continued through each step while three of us sweated away. Finally, David was taking us through verbally as we gingerly began doffing, first palming off the visor. Next was the 0.5% chlorine wash followed by pinching our hoods back. More 0.5% chlorine bleach washing and removal of the hair net. Still another washing, then pulling our zipper tab back and unzipping, pulling our arms through the sleeves to remove the outer gloves as we pulled away, then shimmying our suits off our shoulders until it was heaped at our boots, finally using our boots to anchor and step out of the suit.

"Now stop right there." David the warm and fuzzy now turned serious. "It only takes 10 viral particles of Ebola to stir an infection. That suit just came out of a hot zone and it's loaded with hundreds of millions of viral particles. At this step, another sprayer will spray down the entire suit once you are out of it and it's on the ground. When he is done, you will pick it up and keep it away from your body. Do not let it touch your clothes. Understand? What did I just say?" We repeated back and he continued, "You pick up that suit like it's dog shit. Like it's dog shit that can kill you and put it in the trash can. And you wash your still gloved hands in the 0.5% bleach. One full minute. Now for the final step of removing your inner gloves, inside out using a finger to roll down the cuff and then using the rest to hook it up and remove without touching the skin."

We followed through on the suit disposal and inner glove doffing after which David then had us walking backward with one foot up for spraying, then the other, and so on until out of the hot zone. Here we would wash and rinse with a milder bleach solution of 0.05% followed by soap and water.

Looking at one another, the three of us could see each other's sweat stains in our armpits, necklines and backs. That was 20 minutes. What was 2 hours going to be like?

David then walked the remaining group through the steps, cajoling and correcting as they went. No one was making a joke out of this, which was reassuring.

Taking a break out on the front porch of the hospital office, surveying the courtyard where a gaggle of men were clustered around an ambulance and shouting, I watched to discern what the excitement was about. After several minutes of pronounced gesturing, a man opened the door to the driver's side and hopped in while a couple of others continued to bark at him. He barked back just as vociferously. What was disorganized, organized, and the men all positioned in the rear of the ambulance, began to push until speed was reached and the driver dropped the ambulance's clutch to jump-start the vehicle. It sputtered and died. More shouting and gesturing, then the driver replaced with another driver, and they repeated the process. This time, enough speed was reached and the clutch drop gave way to a running, mobile ambulance that left out the front gate. I wondered who would want their survival to depend on whether or not the ambulance could be push started. No one, but you go with what you have and this is what counted as emergency services.

Back inside the office, the group was in chairs. Mary followed me through the door and plopped down a box, zipping off the tape then handing out phones with instructions on how to use them, where to find our numbers and to program each others' numbers in to our address books. Most of the others had smart phones that they were able to convert or use on the wireless hotspots our employer provided, or they were usable on the Sierra Leone cell system. My phone was a burner and I found it too much of a hassle to get the unlock codes, set up a new account and all that other gibberish so Mary's company phones filled the bill for me. With it, we could make calls to anyone, anywhere there was coverage.

Dr. Thiede called us back to attention. Tomorrow we would go to the Maforki Ebola Treatment Unit for a tour and walk through in our PPE gear. Kati would lead the tour while he remained at the office trying to get the government hospital back on its feet by inventorying supplies, assessing staff levels and otherwise determining what was needed when and where. Questions to David about the challenges he faced in doing this yielded not a lack of knowhow by national staff but reliable inventory, laboratory and diagnostic equipment for them to work with, along with the always ever present conundrum of stable funding. When I told David what I saw with the ambulance in the courtyard and wondered out loud was, "Do they have a trained EMT service and are the ambulances generally reliable, with what I saw being the exception?"

Thiede glanced at his untied shoe, scratched his stubble, then looked at me, chuckling, "Yes. What you saw was an exception. Them being able to start the ambulance at all is actually sort of surprising. Good to hear they got it running because I thought it was completely dead."

With a thud, it landed in my mind that his hands were full beyond anything I imagined. But if you think about it, what good is a running ambulance when all it could do is deliver a patient to what is a hospital in name only. The doctor may or may not be there to direct care and, even if he was, he might not even have tape, suture thread or bandages. Most of us probably have more tape in our homes than the hospital did at that point and time. It was almost like something out of the Civil War where bandages were washed and reused. I was afraid to ask if they recycled needles, not sure if it would be insulting to ask such a question, or if it might be just one other item where it's best to not know-- and if you did, not to say too much.

Dr. Thiede went through our Ebola handouts and covered the history of the disease and current treatment protocols, emphasizing that much of what we were going to be doing would be correct today and probably wrong tomorrow due to the rapid evolution of our understanding. At this juncture, we were to be engaged in what is emergent care, which is we would be treating the acutely ill with all current resources. The hope was that soon there would be more people trained to educate the public on safe techniques regards suspected Ebola cases, contact tracing and other prevention measures.

The afternoon ended and we walked back to our guesthouse, all of maybe 400 yards, which was now simply known as The Ghetto. The goats and dogs certainly didn't mind our appearance in their neighborhood, nor did the hen chickens and chicks who scratched about the side of the road in the knee-deep concrete gutters, extra wide and deep to handle the monsoon rains. All the residents looked and waved while the children would shout, "Apatow! Apatow!" running up to quickly touch us, then running away, cackling and laughing. We certainly stood out, our pale white skin contrasted to their deep ebony.

We arrived back to be greeted by several workers who had come in early November. These were the people who were first to arrive and lend their hands and skills, so it was no surprise to see traces of weariness and battle fatigue in their faces. Immediately, a nurse with a deep French accent and perfect grammatical English who hailed from the Seattle area assaulted our group. Francie's thin shape belied her confidence, something she was not short on I came to believe, with good reason, since she challenged herself to understand and learn. Brett, Kelli and Patti, all nurses, came out to welcome us. Over supper, we learned their resumes, what counted as home, with Washington and Oregon being the best represented with the rest of us from scattered places of the Deep South, Mountain West, New England or Midwest.

The evening wore on and what we were hearing from the Frontier Four repetitively was, "You'll understand by the end of tomorrow what we're up against." Our exchange was natural and spontaneous as if we knew one another for years. We newbies were curious and anxious to get into the thick of it, following on their heels a path they essentially blazed from virgin frontier.

Off the concrete step of the Ghetto porch, a small tan and white dog stretched himself out on top the sand pile beneath the water pump spout, oblivious to us wagging our tongues. Diesel fumes wafted in and out of sense as the generator was now running for the night, giving us lights for the outdoor picnic. Some wandered away to make calls to home via Skype or Facebook to let their families know how things were sifting out thus far, while others stepped outside the front gates to take in the stars and moon of the equatorial sky. Fruit bats flew back and forth, echo locating the bugs attracted by our night-lights. One every once in a time, would swoop inches away from a head then pull away fractions of a second away before impact. Ebola reservoirs with wings, I thought.

I walked into our common area and heard the hum of the freezer and the wop-wop of the generator keeping up. Beer, soda, water and some food items were still tepid to the touch after not cooling all day. I marked two 1.5-liter bottles with my name and took one other into my room with me, unlocking my door latch that was a lock in name only. Going through my luggage, I unpacked scrubs for the next day and rolled out a sheet and blanket I'd packed, my bed for the next 6 weeks beneath a mosquito net that I quickly decided was more of an annoyance, so I wrapped it up over the bed. Otherwise, why the Malerone, right?

Two buckets sat outside my door of about 4 gallons each, put there by our caretakers whenever I put out the empty. I lifted both in and walked them to the bathroom. My nightly ritual of wash and brush was now me kneeling on the floor as I splashed myself with cup after cup of water over my head, shampooing myself and repeating the process cup after cup with a rinse down. I used bottled water for oral hygiene and was able to stand over the sink. One bucket was left over to use for flushing to help me deal with my medical liability. I have no colon but avoided an ileostomy, like my father has, a man who heroically adjusted to his surgical conclusion of ulcerative colitis. Surgical construction resolved my case by using the distal small intestine for a waste reservoir but now I require frequent bathroom breaks.

The one light in my room was dim so I removed the cover to brighten things up. The space was warm and I had a window but thought better to open it for the night since I was sans net, that and the screen was torn. The outlets were all square pegged 220v DC outlets and I popped into the outlet my 110v AC converter to plug in my phone and computer to charge, then set the alarms on both for 6:20 AM. I was ready for sleep; any issues I had with jet lag were nonexistent, though there being only 5 hours time difference between home and Maforki was certainly a plus for maintaining usual rhythms. I laid my head down and realized that my first 24 hours in Sierra Leone was complete. In 12 hours, I was going live as a practicing hospital Ebola nurse working with live people, trying to get them home.

■■

On the Job

Awakening 10 minutes before the phone alarm went off, I pulled back the curtain and let the buttery morning light wash the purple sleep from my eyes. Through the window you could hear the sounds of others rustling about for breakfast and coffee out on the patio deck. Tigger, the compound dog, barked once and someone hushed him. I pulled on fresh scrubs, washed, and then checked my school bag for room key, ID, laptop and incidentals of pen, paper and camera before heading out to the patio for breakfast.

The crew was rummaging about the fixings for hard-boiled eggs, cereals, milk, coffees, teas, breads, spreads, cantaloupe and plantains, a type of African banana. I took my turn, keeping patient for the day's instruction. The Frontier Four of Kelli, Francie, Brett and Patti finished up and packed their work sacks and selves into the minivan Ibrahim just finished washing, the one we arrived in the day before with the rear window sticker of a man with a club chasing stick people, reading, "No one cares about your stick family." Universal humor.

With everyone caffeinated and sated, Kati and Antonino gathered us up for the short walk to the government hospital for some final orientation and instruction review of yesterday's material. The curious eyes of the neighborhood followed us as we clomped past and around the wet potholes of the red gravel road and into the government hospital compound. Dr. Thiede was waiting, looking like he hadn't slept well at all.

We seated ourselves and Dr. Thiede welcomed us, informing us Kelli would be leading our morning walk through Maforki ETU, explaining the reason for the change in plan, saying, "I have to fly out later today back to home...well, what's left of home."

"Everything not OK?" the Major asked, concerned.

Thiede paused, then confessed, "No, I'm afraid not. I got a call last night that our house burned to the ground. Total loss. I have to go home and deal with the clean up and everything else that goes with it. Good news is no one was at home and no one was hurt. I have to get back to deal with the mess."

There was a brief silence followed by our sympathies. For a person who just had 60 years of the belongings of life reduced to a pile of ash, he was being rather philosophical about it, I thought. I could only imagine that maybe the enormity of the situation hadn't quite taken hold yet, and probably wouldn't, until he visited the site of his family tragedy. The family heirlooms, documents, records, photos, maybe your son's lock of hair from his first haircut or a daughter's baby tooth, that letter from the woman you married and your wedding album, or your dad's honor flag that draped his coffin before he was interred along with the quilt your mom made for one of the kid's beds--erased by flame. The helplessness felt by any one of us is what makes us desperate for omnipotence, a way to return time and avert such traumas. The benefit of hindsight is understanding, but the equally galling aspect is learning how impotent we are to repair tragedy.

Dr. Thiede left to take care of his return plans and Kati took over. "We're going to review what we went over yesterday. Everyone gather up all your PPE gear and don. After that, I'll walk you through the doffing process one more time."

We unpackaged all our gear and donned, checking one another out for breaches. The Major returned us to a sense of humor with one of his military days quotes, "Hey, how hard can it be?" goading us all into understanding that maybe we were in over our heads but just didn't know it yet. Like he said, it wasn't pessimism that got the Donner Party into trouble but excessive optimism: 'Sure, we can make it over 'dem mountains 'fore it snows shut.' One winter and 20 shy of what they started out with, the Donners knew better after the fact.

Kati walked us through the doffing, all seven choreographed, WHO approved steps. Satisfied with our performance and that she could keep a safe eye on us all, we loaded into vehicles for the drive down to the Maforki ETU on the outskirts of town, a mile or so distant, with our driver performing the obligatory honking at pedestrians, goats and dogs.

We exited the vehicles into warm sun and a precipitous ditch where two of us stumbled on the loose gravel and surfed to the bottom. Other than learning we needed to watch our steps, the first item that stood out was the blue tarp fence eight feet high that surrounded the complex and the police presence. The other authority figures were two young men, members of the Sierra Leonean military, AK-47's loaded with 30 shot clips strapped over their shoulders. Each person we passed on the way to the nurse's station greeted us enthusiastically, welcoming us to Sierra Leone. Inside the nurses' station, we were shown the day's admissions and team assignments laid out on the whiteboard, each patient with their own tag containing name, age, lab number and date of admission. I counted 34 patients in Suspect and Confirmed. The file system consisted of accounting books listing admissions, deaths and successful discharges. The death book was certainly the most used, its binder cracked and cover much handled. The entire electronic system for record keeping was a laptop, home version printer and one phone for incoming calls of new admissions and outgoing calls to various facilities that handled patient transport and placement, including two local orphanages whose services were needed as the Ebola crisis plodded on.

Strewn about the floor was red dust and paper, the garbage cans already overflowing with discarded food, plastic wraps and prescription medicine boxes. Windows were wide open because where there was supposed to be windows, they were simply open with only a Roman blind to block the elements. Was I surprised? No. I expected basic and comparatively primitive and this was it.

Kati marched us over to the admissions area where an intake national nurse was filling out a brief questionnaire. The patient was then given an admission packet and assigned a room in one of the six Suspect Unit's concrete buildings. Later, a blood draw would be tested for malaria and Ebola. As of now, the turnaround time was 3-4 days, meaning someone with only a fever, criteria enough to get a person admitted, was now in close contact with probable Ebola patients within the confines of the ETU, a Catch-22 hazard we couldn't seem to minimize at this point. However, ideas were already brewing on how to minimize this exposure by dividing the highly likely from the unlikely Ebola infected, further classifying their symptoms as wet or dry. A wet patient would be someone who was active with diarrhea, vomiting and a fever of 101.4 or greater. Additionally, weakness, fatigue and known/suspected contact with a diagnosed Ebola patient in the last 21 days would be considered. A dry patient would be someone who presented with a fever 101.4 but no diarrhea, vomiting or bleeding plus unknown recent Ebola contacts. Malaria, by signs and symptoms, mimics Ebola signs and symptoms. The only way to differentiate the two is by blood work. In the midst of an infectious disease crisis that had captured the world's attention, it was determined that excess caution was the better route, that suspicion was the better option unless you had some known non Ebola reason for your fever and malaise to avoid ending up in a high risk contact environment. On top of that, we were sending the Ebola negative patients home after several days of being in close proximity with positive patients. The only solution to this conundrum would be private rooms and no other human contact but this was simply impossible at this point and time.

As Kati continued speaking, everyone's eyes were taking in the patients sitting on the concrete porches outside the red and white buildings, buckets strewn around the commons area. Minister birds were swooping in and pecking through the garbage for morsels, then flying out and away with other Minister birds taking chase, trying to get them drop whatever treasure the other possessed.

We went out to the perimeter again and plodded down the path past the police post and in through the gate. "Stop!" A diminutive older man ordered, his smile as big as his head. He raised a spray bottle. "Left foot up. Now the right foot please. Thank you." Ali then took us over to the .05% bleach bucket, demonstrated the stubborn spigot and how we needed to wash our hands, a ritual performed countless times a day right up until we left. Last, he pulled out an infrared thermometer, having us present our temple or forehead. All clear, Kati led us into the other nurses' station that was surrounded by a beehive of activity under silver tin roof canopies that stretched the length of sidewalks going to the other buildings. Behind our station was the national nurses' station and next to that was the Cuban medical detail's workspace. Across the way was the administrative building of the national nurse Matron, Rebecca, a large tired looking woman, and ETU director and native, Dr. George, a gregarious man who welcomed us warmly.

Inside our station, the floor had its share of detritus and personal belongings of its users strewn about, book bags and notebooks tucked into every corner. The ceiling fan hummed overhead, keeping it pleasant. The drone of the generator in the background was a constant.

Kati took one of the empty seats and we did the same. She instructed us that we would be following the four veterans on their second pass through the unit but that we would not be performing any patient care. "I want you to just watch. Ask questions, but try not to get in the way. It's hot today and they'll probably only be able to stay in for about 90 minutes. Get yourself some water and drink up now, then we'll go over to the supply room to get fitted for boots."

With water in hand, Kati had us dodge over to the supply room to confront piles of boxes with black marker scribbling that indicated what was more or less in each mound. The person in charge of inventory seemed bothered, that we would need something from him, but he complied, dug through the boxes until he came to the boots, asking our sizes and trying to pull out our lucky number, mine being ten. When we left, the warehouseman didn't seem much concerned about the disarray created and turned his back on the jumble he'd created in securing our boots.

Back at the nurses' station, Kati handed out finger nail polish she pulled from a desk drawer that was a drawer in name only, as it stuck and had to be jiggered every which way. The others found duct tape to put around the boot cuff and marker their names on. I decided the unique way to ID my own boots was not with initials but with a sideways 8, the symbol for infinity, and, no, there was no special deep meaning attached to this, just that it was unique and hopefully would prevent my boots from being used by someone else.

As we poked through the drawers and cabinets, waiting for our turn to go inside, I noticed silence. Then I noticed the nice breeze abated. Generator rest period time. And at the warmest part of the day no less.

Outside the two hundred or so national workers were jostling, laughing and arguing in Krio and English under the shade of the trees, coming by in twos and threes to catch a glimpse of us through the open door. If any of us had any question on what the attraction was, it was answered then and it was us.

Patti, Kelli, Francie and Brett could be heard bantering outside with the nationals after exiting the dining hall where they had lunch. Residual sweat stained their scrubs, red dust covered their tennis shoes, hopeless to keep them clean. You could see the heat in their faces and the matching mouse nests of hair manufactured by the morning bustle. Patti, with her straight blonde Scandinavian hair defying mouse nest description, was betrayed by her fired up complexion expressing the day's heat.

"You guys ready for the big tour," Brett smirked. "Back home you'd have to pay to see this; here you get to see it for free."

"Don't scare them away now," Francie admonished. "Let's get a couple weeks out of them first."

Kelli was quiet. Watching her, you knew she took what she did seriously and wanted us to do the same. Every group needs that person, the one who parses between the best that can be done and when to ignore the nonsense that got in the way of doing the job. I had no intention of disappointing her and decided I would follow her lead, not that the other three weren't as capable, because they were. However, there is always that one person you view as your superior, whose opinion matters more for reasons that are as much an enigma as our own personalities and characters are to others, even ourselves. Yes, she was a pediatric nurse, about as far away from my own background as you could get, and the Major with his pediatric background made the two a natural fit. In general, one grasped Kelli had a hold on what worked in these conditions.

"Get a good, cold drink into you. Make sure to write your name on your water bottle," Brett advised. "Bathrooms are down at the end of the walkway, so make sure you use it before suiting up. No watches, jewelry or anything else. Anything you take inside stays inside. You're the only thing that comes out."

Kati led us to the donning station to boot up, gathering up suits, gloves, visor and masks off the shelf. Each of us wrapped ourselves into our white Tyvek, masked and gloved, placed our aprons and had a national tie us in snug. With red markers in hand, the nationals asked our names, pronouncing them twice and asking us for the spelling, then writing our name on the front of our apron followed by our shoulder and back. Donned, we were all identical so the moniker was important. The sprayers, who carried the 30 pounds of 0.5% solution on their backs, did the same. In all, on any given go-in to the hot zone, there could easily be 40 people ranging from sprayers following all staff to continuously disinfect, to the national nurse or nurses assigned to each expatriate group to translate between patients and us expats.

We bumped each other's elbows to show readiness and the national staff gave us a visual once over and approval. Kati mother-ducked all of us ducklings into line and led the way in, reminding us that once we passed through the upcoming gate, under no circumstances could we turn back.

The first gate was technically on hinges, but by any building code standard they were useless, so Kati had to lift and push to open the gate. "Watch for the sharp edges on the latches. These gates are real whores." She went ahead of us and patiently waited until the last one was through and pushed the gate back shut. Each of us had several 1.5-liter bottles to distribute to the patients for their hydration. Our simple job was to encourage them to drink to replace the copious amounts of fluids they were losing to diarrhea and vomiting.

First approach was to the six buildings in the Suspect Unit numbered 1-6. Outside on the porches, some of the patients milled about, appearing by all accounts relatively healthy, awaiting their laboratory results to see if they were Ebola or malaria positive. One could easily surmise that these patients, up of their own volition and power, were most likely negative and had the misfortune of being caught in the Ebola net that deemed all temperatures over 101.4 be treated as potential positive and quarantined here.

We crossed over the gravel courtyard and into the first building. Garbage was overflowing from the one garbage can in an open room where bars hemmed in the windows and bare concrete floors sweated out the rainy season humidity. The beds were 4 feet off the ground, without safety rails and had a hole in the center where a patient could place their buttocks and a diarrhea catch bucket beneath caught the involuntary explosions from the patient's bowels as they crapped themselves into hypovolumic shock. Several full buckets were scattered toward the center of the room and more than enough excrement and puke were in various spots on the floor. Three patients were on their beds, in their street clothes soaked throughout from their own bile. Kati approached the first one, handled the wrist of the patient to read the name on the wristband and introduced herself. "Wata," she said, offering one of the bottles we brought in with us. "Important you drink. OK?"

The patient, a shirtless young woman of 20 years, her lips caked with yellow snot, wordlessly peered back at us through her blood shot eyes and took the bottle. Kelli cracked the cap and helped hold the bottle up to the woman's lips. She was not eager to drink but did take in small sips and after several minutes of maybe half going into her and the other half dribbling down her cheeks and neck, she waved us off. Visibly exhausted and her breathing labored, she hiccupped twice then regurgitated the water over the side of the bed. Nearby, her Styrofoam lunch carton of rice and fish was untouched and her breakfast was face down on the floor with ants working it over. The woman continued to hiccup and Kelli gently pulled the dry portion the woman's lafa over her torso.

Dr. Galleo stated the obvious, "Is there any chance we can start IV fluids on her soon?" Galleo was direct to the point in his tone but he was correct. Without supplemental hydration, this woman did not stand a chance and soon enough her electrolytes would be, and probably already were, wildly out of normal. Shock would follow as her red blood cells exploded, diminishing her ability to transport basic life supporting oxygen to her tissues. Potassium and sodium, necessary for proper nervous system function, would not be present in the right ratios and her autonomic systems such as respirations and heart rate, would first likely race to compensate for systemic acidosis, then crash and eventually arrest. During all this, her lungs would likely fill with fluid as lung tissue ruptured, accompanied by some bleeding that might be evident around her mouth and eyes, the worst manifestations of the Ebola virus. As if she didn't have enough to deal with, she likely was dealing with opportunistic secondary infections normally kept at bay in a healthy body but which could now bloom since her white cell count, necessary for battling infections, was likely in the basement.

Kati sighed, "We're still waiting on IV needles. We have the solution and tubing. From what I heard last night, the only available IV needles are non-safety IV needles. We'd like to have the safety needles because the last thing we want is someone to get stuck trying to place an IV."

Galleo nodded, but I knew he wasn't going to accept that. "Is there any type of charting going on so that when we see each patient we can review what has and hasn't been done?"

"Not yet; we still need to put together a sheet we can bring in and leave in here. They think it should be laminated," Kati offered.

"Laminated? We just put them on clipboards and hang them on the end of the bed." Galleo was hostile to these hurdles for the simple reason that at this stage of the game, anything would be an improvement. Any waiting for perfection was wasting time and energy that could be devoted to more therapeutic care.

"They're worried about patient privacy, that the other patients might read them." Kati was not defending the current system but merely mouthing the objections of the 'They'.

'They' is that entity that exists in some unknown room typing out email memos why something shouldn't or should be done, oblivious to the real life ramifications of over rationalizing ideas into uselessness. It is the third great force of the universe behind gravity and light. It exists, but is nearly impossible to measure, to define its beginning or its end. Yet, it crushes as an implosion stretched over periods of time that outlasts any human interest in challenging it.

Galleo's response crescendoed, "They're all here for suspected or confirmed Ebola. I hardly think this is any great secret the patients aren't keeping from each other or anyone else."

Kati demurred, "You're right. We'll talk about it when we get outside. Time to move on. We aren't supposed to be doing patient care on this round, just hand out water to those who need it."

We left Suspect 1 and moved across the courtyard to the double gates separating Suspect units from the Confirmed units. The blue tarp fencing was nailed to stick-logs, the nails bent over, rusty and sharp. Our sprayer, an anonymous set of eyes peering from behind a mask and visor, identifiable only by his name of "Racin" scrawled across his apron, demanded, "Stop. Hands out." Here we all stopped and placed our hands in front of us and Racin sprayed, instructing "Rub and wash," in his Krio accent. He pumped his bleach pack several times to maintain pressure of the spray, making certain each hand was washed before misting our boots, fronts and legs.

Spraying done, Kati led us through the double gates and onto the Confirmed landing. I could see in what showed of her face, around her eyes, that she was flush. I knew she wasn't going to complain, either. "How are you all doing? A little warm? Wouldn't it be great if sex were always this hot." She was in fine spirits per the usual.

My own body temperature was warmer than normal and I could feel the socks in my boots sopping up. After decades running in high summer heat, I had a firm grasp of my own physiological limits. A healthy body compensates for physical assault in a number of ways. With heat it is sweat on the skin that evaporates to create a cooling. Our capillaries near the skin surface dilate, creating a flush look, to dissipate heat, and our respirations grow deeper to help throw off excess heat just as dog does by panting. In its own way, you become comfortable with the perspiration when it's expected.

The Frontier Four were methodically going patient to patient through the Confirmed units, each one with a national nurse and sprayer to form a team and take on one building each. We entered the tin roofed and tarped buildings, the builder in me couldn't help but assess the structural integrity. These were not the professionally built concrete buildings of the Suspect units, abandoned trade school classrooms, but a quickly thrown together project. The trusses did not have a continuous bottom chord. Wherever they fell short in the span between walls, the chords were simply plated together with an additional piece where they fell short, causing a sag. Snow weight limits certainly were of no concern in this part of the world, but you wouldn't want to be walking on the roof with too many people for whatever reason. Just as interesting, I could see the rafters were not fortified and braced symmetrically, spaced about 10 feet apart, a concession to the amount of materials the carpenters had to work with. A hard rain with some wind might have been enough to undo the truss work with injurious consequences for any hapless soul beneath.

We placed ourselves in the center of the room, observing as a medical team cared for each patient. Patients were in their beds trying to rest and quietly wish away the discomfort. The more critically ill were on the floors, possibly to cool their fevers—or a cultural predilection of sleeping on the ground. We could only speculate, but Kati saw this as a sign that death was imminent. The cholera beds themselves with the aperture in the middle were not an item of comfort either, as much an object of inconvenience as if there was a stump in the middle of the bed.

We walked to the next building, stepping over uneaten rice and fish spilled on the ground, half empty water bottles rolling amidst human waste soaked clothes. Several patients were sprawled across the front walkway and didn't flinch as we stepped over them, either not caring or not knowing. One middle aged gentleman was at the water faucet, rinsing himself down, and by all accounts was past the worst of the disease, now waiting on blood work to confirm if his viral count was low enough for him to be released home, a near miraculous accomplishment that warranted a small celebration when it happened.

Our 90 minutes were finished. Kati led us to the doffing station, another haphazard construction project of unevenly poured concrete, corrugated tin roofing, various pieces of lumber and sticks nailed and tied to together wrapped up in blue nylon tarp. Though none of us other than Kati had touched an infected patient, the amount of bodily fluids from the patients smeared across floors, walkways and gates, likely had Ebola lurking at the absolute least on the leggings and boots of our suits. The protocol doffing began with us watching Kati go through the process to refresh our memories.

Each one of us took our turn. First, having our hands sprayed and rubbing them for one minute, then transitioning to spread eagle with the sprayer misting us neck down, front to back. We each then had our boots sprayed down, employing the one legged hop for each boot bottom. Several were ahead of me so I had to wait my turn. I found myself anxious to get out of the suit and mask for a breath of cool, fresh air. Soon enough, my turn came and I was sprayed down. My next move was to step into a tub of 0.5% bleach solution and slosh my boots about for another minute. My eyes burned from the bleach solution fumes, reminder enough you did not want this concentration on your skin. It was more comfortable to hold my breath in fits and starts, to avoid irritating my throat and lungs anymore than need be. On to the bucket and another washing of the hands for one minute before palming off my visor into a waiting tub of bleach, then another minute of washing hands. Next was to detab the zipper, zip down and pull back the hood. Now for the shimmy down, trying to worm the suit off past the boots while simultaneously retrieving the arms inside out, letting the wrist tabs peel back the outer layer of gloves. This resulted in more contortions than I cared to count, but eventually both boots and gloves were through the worst bottleneck of the process. Again, another minute of hand washing followed by removing the N-95 mask, carefully pinched with two fingers at the mask front point, then pulled back in one motion to let the rubber band take the hair net off. In the meantime, a sprayer at the end of the walk was spraying down my suit with my back to the process as he instructed. With everything off and the doffed suit sprayed to the sprayers satisfaction, he had me pick it up, where I then bent over with one thought running through my mind, 'Pick it up and hold it away from you like it's dog crap that can kill you'. I did, holding it out arms' length, depositing it in a garbage can as if it were nuclear waste. Another minute of hand washing and I carefully degloved my hands, taking pains not to touch the skin of my arms. Finally, the walk backwards doing the one legged hop with boot bottom to the sprayer. "Right. Left. Right again. Left again. Good. Wash up over there." The .05% solution felt good on my arms, diluting the 0 .5% bleach solution that leaked down into my gloves and settled on my wrists, irritating the skin. Soap and water followed with a thorough scrub of the arms and one final rinse. My entire scrub outfit was soaked with not a single dry spot, my hair wet enough to shake out heavy drops of sweat.

Outside the doffing station, I waited for the others to come through and each looked as wet and hot as the next person did. Other ETU workers were milling about under the shade of the tree, taking the required breaks from being in the PPE whether they were nurses, cleaners, sprayers or burial team members. The late afternoon call to prayer went out not in the stereotypical way of a sound system belting out the call, but a man simply reminding his fellow Muslim worshippers it was that time of day and off they shuffled into an open space, going down to their prayer rugs, kneeling and facing east towards Mecca.

No drama to our walk-about as intended. It was clear that the number of patients to nurses and doctors was seriously out of kilter and that the addition of us would be a huge step forward in providing a higher level of care. The discussion at the supper table would be interesting and I looked forward to hearing what the docs had in mind for improvements and how the division of labor would shake out.

Back at the nurses' station, we all grabbed cool waters from the freezer and the generator was up and running again, giving us back the ceiling fan to help dry us out. It was good to get out of the boots and back into tennis shoes. Our drivers shouted from the gates that it was time to go back to the Ghetto so we all loaded up, sweaty and dusty, looking forward to supper. I soon learned that supper looked forward to us as well.

■■

On Our Own

After our return to the Ghetto, we all bucket washed and changed into nice, dry clothes. Our guardians Chris and Nolan had arranged for supper to greet us every night, spread out on the patio picnic tables, buffet style. Salad fixings of vegetables, cucumber, tomato, lettuce, papaya, plantains and oranges were on one plate accompanied by some sort of pilaf dish peppered with vegetables while the main course was in surprise-of-the-day tins where one would find the evening selection. Tonight it was a whole fish on white rice. The fish, with its eye in place but not intact, dehydrated and sunk into the skull, didn't look much different than a crappie I'd find three days old on a Wisconsin lake shoreline. It was good. With enough of any sauce of one's taste, mine being hot n' spicy out of a bottle, it satisfied. Anyways, who was I to criticize the cooks who put this together. For all I knew, they spent the better part of a day preparing the cooked portions over a wood-fueled fire, not a comfortable occupation in the warmer parts of the world.

The three doctors quizzed the Frontier Four over dinner and drinks well into the evening, a back and forth of trying to ascertain what was available, what was being done and what we could do, starting in the morning, to drop the abysmal 90% Maforki ETU mortality rate. The rest of us watched and listened, letting the medical hierarchy take its natural course, with the three docs taking the lead. The decision was made that the Major and Kelli would focus their pediatric talents and experience on the pediatric patients, a chance pairing that could do nothing but help. Listening to the Major's occasional anecdotes about his own seven children, several he and his wife adopted out of foster care, pediatrics was a natural fit where he had some emotional skin in the game. Galleo and Peterson were adamant about finding ways to get more fluids going on the patients, as well as working with the Frontier Four's idea that treating secondary infections would offer patients a better chance at overcoming their primary Ebola infection.

The bats were out, doing their back and forth under the one light we had. The one beer I had was tugging me to rack in for the night. A couple of others had wandered off to their rooms as well. When I went to bed, I could hear the soft conversations continuing. The room was a bit stifling so I turned on my own fan and opened the bathroom window to bring in the cooler night air. As I cleaned up, a visitor appeared on the window's side casement, a little bookii house gecko who felt he deserved to be just about anywhere his four legs could carry him, including the walls I discovered, as he scampered in and up into the corner of the bathroom.

I watched him. He watched me. Was it worth the effort to try to catch him? No. If I tried, he'd bolt who knows in which direction and I'd be spending half the night trying to get him out of the room. However, I had to try, otherwise I'd be spending the night waiting for him to make the right move. When I reached my hand up to corner him, he zipped right back to the open window. Happy he was out in the wild again, I slammed the window, glad that chore was completed, or I was glad until I saw about a ½ inch green tip of a tail that was caught in the window and cut off. Thinking he might still be attached, I reopened the window to see the curious lizard apparently ambivalent about losing that part of his tail since he exhibited no fear that I could discern. If he was OK, I was OK. Bedtime.

Morning breakfast was the typical picking over of breads, spreads and jams, everyone vying for the coffee at the same time. I took the opportunity to pocket a couple of eggs for the walk to the ETU.

Some had decided to walk and I decided to do the same, knowing it would be a good chance to see the town on a more personal level. It was now predictable that the kids would be running up to us shouting, "Apatow", and they did. The one fat woman in the city was at her deep fry cooking fire placing dough into her pot and laying out a crudely formed doughnut into baskets. Three for 500 Leones was fair enough and she handed the product over, her children excited that Apatow were doing business with the family. Dogs approached, but not to be fed so much as simply acknowledged. Tigger stuck to our heals for the first half mile or so and the other dogs seemed to sense that we belonged to Tigger, thus their interest was just in passing and they left us alone. None had any collars, tags or any evidence of ownership, let alone vaccinations or other veterinary care. I reflected that forgoing a rabies vaccine before leaving now looked like a poor idea even though the dogs displayed no overt aggression. Out of literally thousands of dogs, there had to be that one or two who weren't so oblivious or indifferent to our presence. I did not want to be the person that found that dog—and I didn't. Keri did.

Keri packed her stash of deep fried doughnuts into her school bag and zipped it shut, no different from anyone else. We all continued walking past the city circle shops and approached the Bankasoka river bridge where the looming hydroelectric skeleton slumbered. Chickens and puppies and kids meandered out of our way as the traffic honked at us in either a 'hello' or 'look out' manner. You never knew which. A couple of brown and tans trotted alongside to keep us company, maybe hoping we'd adopt them or treat them. Then the spine-wrenching scream pierced the air and out off the gravel driveway going up into the dam construction site, a mutt bolted and leapt in full snarl, sinking its teeth into Keri's bag. With one screeching and the other snarling, a fight to the death tug of war started until Keri thought better of it and dropped the bag, running to the center of road. A Land Rover and two motorcycles dodged her and several others stopped, trying to comprehend the theatrical white lady, a former college basketball player and veteran African medical worker who more than could handle herself. As Keri regrouped, her shocked expression folding into one of determined revenge and to reclaim her bag, the dog dropped the bag and approached. Fast. Before either could bite or kick the other, four men came running into the street from their front yards on the road, with one handling a stick and another a red rock in hand. The dog was quickly overwhelmed, went back on its haunches and turned tail but took two snaps at the other two unarmed saviors before doing so. Surrounded, the man with the stick lifted it high over his head and let it crash towards the animal's skull as the other simultaneously threw his rock. The stick hit the blacktop, splintering, and the rock at best grazed the dog's belly, putting a small gouge into the road surface. As quick as it all started, the dog was off down the riverbank and into the brush.

"What's wrong with the fucking dog!," Keri spit out. The four men, speaking all at once, surrounded Keri with one of them handing her bag back, two small tears sunk through the nylon corner. Her breathing slowed back down and by the time the rest of us even knew something was happening, the whole incident was over. With profuse 'thank yous' from Keri to her four rescuers, and the four seemingly very happy with their contribution to salvaging Keri's hide, they returned to their day with the next few minutes devoted by all to recreating the story and processing the motive of the dog. It had to be the doughnuts was the consensus. I was thinking, 'rabies', but kept it to myself as my guess was exactly no more than that, a guess. Besides, rabies isn't a disease known for pack organization.

With the morning excitement past, we continued to work. The usual spray your feet wash your hands protocol ensued as we entered and ducked into our nurse's station for the morning plan. A thin young man, national nurse Martin, came in and welcomed us. Going to the grease board, he asked our attention then went down the names, delivering his memorized notes on each patient's condition, lab results for Ebola and malaria, anticipated discharges and any overnight mortality. Rumor had it that he had not had a day off since the outbreak in Port Loko last August and his tired presentation seemed to back that up.

After the morning report, we searched our team assignment and all of us newbies were divided amongst the four veterans along with one national nurse to each team. The three doctors went over to the supply room and came back with bags of IV fluid and IV needles while others gathered up oral rehydration salt packets, ORS, to mix into the 1.5 liter bottles that we'd distribute to the patients to keep their electrolytes up. These two items were the product of the previous night's discussion and with the new added work force, it would be easier to implement the new therapies. In one day, the Maforki ETU was going from about 24 nurse/doctor hours per day to 96 man-hours.

10 a.m. arrived and all the teams descended on the donning tent. A flurry of packaging littered the floor in two minutes as we stuffed and taped ourselves in and the nationals tied and inked us up for our entry. Brett led our team along with Dorine, a national nurse who'd interpret and fill us in on other crucial cultural dos and don'ts. Galleo and I would follow behind. Our wards would be the Suspect Units 1-4 which held about 15 patients who may or may not have moved during the night between buildings.

Already the heat was making us sweat through the scrubs. Everyone was visibly flushed around the eyes. Just as we finished filing through the first gate, someone let out an 'Ow!' followed by a cuss. Gwyn had attempted to move the gate back a bit further to give us more room but scraped her wrist along one of the sharp metal edges of the latch, tearing open her glove and peeling her skin back about 3 inches with some slight red oozing. "Stop. Don't go any further," Kelli commanded. "No one touch her."

You could see the disappointment in Gwyn's eyes. Barely a foot into the hot zone she was done and over. Kelli and the Major approached to examine while Gwyn held up her left wrist. Kelli empathized, "I'm so sorry, Gwyn. You have to stay out at least for today and probably a couple of days until that heals. You touched nothing other than the gate, right?"

Gwyn concurred, "No, just the gate. Do I go all the way through or backtrack?"

Kelli looked at the boundaries set up and made the smarter decision. "You aren't in the hot area. Close, but not in. Anyways, it would just be risky to have you walk all the way through known infected areas to the doffing station. You're still clean but we'll have the sprayer mist you right here, boot to hood, and you doff right here. Go back to the nurse's station and we'll talk when I come out. OK, girlie?"

"OK." Gwyn slightly nodded. "See you when outside."

"Heads up on those sharp objects everyone," Brett reminded us. From that moment on, I knew that the need for constant vigilance was the single most important thing I could do.

Dorine, Brett and I rubbed our way down the walkway to Suspect, our PPE swishing away. Carrying a biohazard bag full of pharmaceutical odds and ends that included Paracetamol for pain control, diazepam for anxiety to help patients relax and sleep through the worst of it, metoclopromide for the nausea and bags of IV fluid and 20 gauge IV needles for those unable to drink enough to ward off dehydration.

Brett led the way in, pushing the heavy metal red door back against the wall. The night wasn't friendly to patients as the floor was littered with vomit, spilled food and full waste buckets. No smell. The sprayers kept any spills bleached to negate infection spread with the added benefit that it stopped the rotting stench that comes from sewage. The plastic table housing our drugs and meager supplies were in disarray and the neat-nic in me wanted to clean the place up but that wasn't our first priority.

Our first patient had no lab results back but it was obvious he was critical as he lay sprawled out on the concrete floor, eyes rolled back in his head and mental state deteriorated. Malaria could do this as well as Ebola but it didn't matter either way until we knew for certain. There was no sense in giving anti-malarials to an Ebola patient since we still didn't have them in great supply, meaning we should only give it when we knew for certain. Either way, he was on his way out.

Brett stepped over him and got down on his knees and looked into the man's eyes, trying to discern how neurologically intact he was at that moment. Dorine, speaking in Krio, asked the man to give his name. No response. Brett pinched the skin on the man's forearm and the patient pulled his arm away, nothing verbal, though his eyes tried to focus, making him a 4 or 5 on a Glasgow scale of 15. The temporal thermometer showed a 39.5 fever, about 103 F. The skin tented, meaning he was severely dehydrated. We thought of putting the man back on his bed, deciding against it since he would likely roll off and fall 4 feet to the concrete, adding blunt force trauma to his travails. Dorine put a bottle to his lips and tried to get water in, but the man's swallow reflex was absent. As soon as his head was not being held, it would flop back to the side and all the water spilled out of his mouth. Brett and I pulled the man from the center of the floor to in between the beds. There Brett bundled up a lafa and placed it under his head. "No, he's not going to be here tomorrow."

I bent over to take a quick look into his eyes and for a second I thought he may have responded to my look but it was fleeting if it did happen. With my Catholic upbringing, I fell back on recalling the movements of the sacrament of Last Rites, crossing his forehead with my finger but sans oil and water used to anoint. It was not the least I could do; it was the most I could do. All of this took about 10 minutes.

What struck me, an American trained nurse, was how we made the decision to continue to treat or not treat this man. Back in the States, no nurse would ever make that call and only a doctor would do such and then only after likely consultation with colleagues, and by all means consulting with family along with referring to any legal directions the patient may have left regards their care, something that not atypically took several days. In a space of a few minutes, we three nurses decided it was over and no further treatment would be useful. No family talk. No ethics board. No lawyers. No attending physician or specialists. Now the man was on the hard concrete and the best we did was a balled up lafa for a pillow.

Off our knees, the sprayer had us hold our hands out and we disinfected. Out next patient had been watching us, a 15 year old girl. Dorine jumped in immediately with Krio questions, asking if she was feeling warm, nauseous, was able to eat and drink, or generally felt well or not. At times the girl's answers were so soft and quiet Dorine had to ask her to repeat herself. I put the scanning thermometer to her forehead and got back a 37.9, which meant she did not meet the fever guideline of 38.5C (101.4F) for admission any longer but that no longer mattered; she was in and there was no out until the lab results came back.

I offered her a bottled water and Brett pointedly directed her to drink, indicating we wanted to witness that she was capable of doing so. The girl looked at Dorine for confirmation, which she did, and the girl took a strong drink, pulling out a ¼ of the bottle. Her food tin was clean, evidencing she was eating well, meaning her PO would be assessed as excellent, sparing her having us jamming around her arm with an IV needle trying to find a vein. The real problem she had was getting out of here uninfected, a tragic Catch-22 where a fever of 39.5 or greater, no matter the origin, had to be assumed to be an Ebola infection, a stark and solid criteria that was throwing Ebola and non-Ebola patients together in our Suspect buildings, creating a high risk situation for the uninfected. In a better hospital, such patients would be put into private rooms and kept from one another to limit contact and spare the misdiagnosed the drama and tragedy of risking their lives waiting for a lab result. No one spoke much of this, yet when I did bring it up later on, the reactions were hard and firm, as if we had no choice in the matter, that it was an issue decided not by us but by the laws of Nature and gravity of it all, therefore beyond our control. At first blush, this seems uncaring and brutal. However, there was no better way available. One could blame money, infrastructure, bureaucrats, nature of the disease, etc., but it was all we had at that moment in time to push back against the spread of the disease. Leaving someone in the community until we knew for absolute certain the cause of a fever would be even more irresponsible as well. 39.5 C had become a number that put people in line, behind a fence, guarded by men with guns, where faceless white suited people with only eyes came to touch them, even then with a thick layer of rubber in between, hardly conducive to establishing a warm relationship. The rights of a nation outweighed the rights of the person. I believe we were enamored of that idea, to protect us from the crushing weight of the unfairness of it all, to those who were uninfected yet thrown into a pen by dint of a thermometer that read 39.5 C. All to fight off an invisible monster.

Her name was Sally Kargbo, the 15 year old with her quiet voice. How she must have laid there at night listening to the wretching others, trying to keep her distance, washing her hands constantly to fend off the germs that could come and get her, hiding for days before she even knew and days more before we would know using science.

Brett patted her on the back and gave her thumbs up for her drinking and eating. He asked Dorine to tell her that we'd be waiting on the lab results and hopefully discharge her to home. Sally simply nodded then eased herself down back onto her cholera bed, looking away.

Our next patients were in various stages of decline and we administered Paracetamol for pain and Valium for the anxiety. For those who could not drink or would not drink, the IV needle was unpackaged and Brett would place it while Dorine or I would hold the arm and release the tourniquet when a patent intravenous strike was made. One of us would hold the bag high to get a good flow then hunt the wall for a place to hang the bag high enough so it could gravity feed while we moved on. On the cinder block walls there was nothing, so the slate glass windows, piece of loose string or twisted up plastic was used as a hanger to fix the bag into a hanging position. With a couple of squeezes we coaxed the bag to empty, hopefully before having to leave so we could hang a second liter of fluids. A month had passed since Brett arrived as one of the other Frontier Four and today, for the first time, he was able to administer IV fluids, the single most important treatment that would give patients a fighting chance by getting as much fluid into themselves as they expelled out, avoiding shock.

After 10 or 11 patients, recharging a couple of IV bags and getting others started, trying to coax the poor drinking patients to take some liquid, along with lifting and positioning them on their beds, the heat of the day was sapping us, making us nothing but bags of fluid ourselves. As a national nurse, Dorine had a strict 90 minute time limit her matron enforced and she was now a half hour over. We finished what we set out to do and 4 hours later we would be back in to check our previous work, tackling any new developments as they presented themselves. Brett called it and we walked our way across the courtyard then through and past the confirmed buildings, noticing those assigned there were still busy with patients more acutely ill as a whole than ours. Everyone was tying up loose ends before heading to the doffing station and getting their daily dose of scorch and scratch, that being the bleach that leaked under the glove cuffs and burned your wrists and the fumes that provoked a cough for many of us, leaving irritated airways.

Back at the nurses' station, Kelli now checked out Gwyn's gouge, giving Gwyn the bad news that not until the scrape closed over could she go back in the hot zone. Now she needed to find another job until she healed and it was her misfortune that turned out to be our good luck when Gwyn took over the admissions/discharge process, a job that assessed arriving patients, got their labs ordered and reported, and arranged for discharged patients to be given food, money, clothes and a taxi home. This involved making phone calls to connect the dots and run things in an orderly flow. Gwyn's clients weren't just the patients coming in and going out but all the other people who brought people in and took people home, including the Catholic Church orphanage and Port Loko social services that would try to help patients integrate back into their villages, a formidable task. Too often people who were in an Ebola hospital were rejected by their home villages, and even their own families were turning away to avoid the associated stigma. Gwyn found the people who were the fixers and put A to B out of an alphabet soup of competing demands with deadlines stacked on deadlines. It was a job where you had to constantly think 6 steps ahead and have 10 different contingencies in place for when step 5 of 6 blew up. Just watching her work was enough to scramble your brains and I doubt I could do the same as she did without pulling out handfuls of hair. We definitely ended up on the better end of the deal, striking gold with Gwyn.

In between a.m. and p.m. rounds, we talked and had lunch with the national nurses. Dorine was my fixer, pointing me in the direction of who to see for what, vouching for me to the Lunch Lady, a portly, dour woman who mentally weighed and measured me and, I suspect, found me wanting. She deemed that I was OK to have one of the delivered lunches, an item where sometimes the numbers came up short and some left out of a meal. If that was the case, the nationals seeing me walk off with a lunch while their colleagues ended up on the short end of the stick would not ingratiate this 54 year old white guy American with the locals.

At 30 years old, Dorine was one of the first of a class of Port Loko trained nurses a few years back and was the only person in her family at this moment to have steady work, making her the breadwinner for her own two kids, husband, mother, father and brother. With 70 or 80% unemployment, jobs at the Ebola unit were desirable and it was routine to find the man spraying boots or on corpse detail was a bi or tri lingual college graduate. I can only guess at Dorine's wages but one thing observed was that many of the nurses were on the heavier side compared to the general population, so the wages were apparently enough to provide for higher quantities of food. Sometimes I'd see the nurses with soda-pops, a nonexistent item in the hands of most other locals. Sweets were high luxury.

It was hot. What else could you say? So just when all of us were dried out it was time to don and go in again. Our team would be escorting an admission in addition to the normal duties we performed. Brett and I went over to the warehouse and rummaged around in a corner for something, anything we could use for rags, clothes or blankets but the pickings were slim and none, leaving us only with rags and not many of those. Now in his fifth week, I sensed Brett was disappointed he couldn't do more for the comfort of the patients but for what he could, he put the best spin on it. Is that a coping method? Just his nature? In any assessment or judgment, people try to perform in the context of the situation, something referred to as relativism, as opposed to idealism where everything fails every single time and makes perfectionism look chancy.

Brett sighed, swinging the bag of rags as we walked back to the donning station, every worker on the site shouting out his name in greeting. I asked, "You know all these fellows? There has to be a couple hundred on the grounds."

"No," was his flat response. "I tried for a few days to learn their names but it seems like all the men are named Muhammad. I can't keep them straight. Some have western names and they seem easier. What's that say, huh?"

"Cultural gap that takes time filling I suppose," I mused. "I've found that with accents it takes my ear awhile to adjust to the nuances. I'm sure they'll think I'm deaf when I keep asking them to repeat something over and over."

As we approached the national nurse tent station, you could hear the gals going back and forth, laughing, picking on one of their own for who knows what. Brett knocked and we were summoned in. They all had cots with clothes hung neatly on racks along with cell phones, laptops or video players that kept them entertained between rounds. Dorine saw us and jumped up to join us.

After the usual flurry of donning amongst 40 odd people in a space you wouldn't rent out to a laying hen, we were ready and headed in with the bottles of ORS water, meds, rags and IV supplies. Brett directed me to cross over the courtyard and go to the fence to check on the admission coming in while he and Dorine went in and started on the patients.

I crossed the rocky courtyard and went to the fence to see who I could scare up at the admissions building and see where the new patient was. Since no one was outside and all inside, I stood at the fence and wailed, "Can someone come out!" Tick-tock, tick-tock, tick-tock and sweat in the sun. I shout a couple of more times and Gwyn appears. "Our admission arrive yet?"

"No," Gwyn responded. "She's coming from about 50 miles away so it could be awhile. We've got two walk-ins out front. Do you know if anybody else is available to take them?"

'Uh-oh', I thought, 'this means 'me'. "Uhm, well, no. I suppose we could take them. They'd be going into suspect, right?"

"Yes."

"Any idea how long before their ready?" I asked.

"Two nationals are donning now and will do the assessment and set them up. All you have to do is come to the admission area when we yell and walk them in," Gwyn instructed.

"Easy enough. Just yell loud so I can hear you inside the buildings. We'll be in Suspect 1-4."

The admission area was a spot in the driveway behind where the ambulance normally unloaded, wet and muddy from water and bleach buckets overflowing and spilling, probably one of the cleanest spots in Africa considering how many gallons of bleach treated water soaked the ground.

Gwyn nudged me out of my thoughts. "Rick, Sally Kargbo, 15. Her labs came back and she's negative-negative. She can go home. Bring her to the shower and then to the fence in back. We'll give her fresh clothes and discharge her. And here are the names of two other labs that tested positive and they need to be escorted over to confirmed," Gwyn rattled off as she handed over a piece of paper with the information all handwritten on notebook paper.

"OK," I responded, trying to sound enthusiastic as my head started sorting out how I would do all this and what it meant for my expected duties. I left the fence and caught up with Brett and Dorine. No sooner did I walk in than Brett gave me an order, pointing to the floor, "He's gone. Go to the fence and get a body bag, please." With that he turned around and continued working on the patient he and Dorine were with, trying to get him to swallow some water and Paracetamol, already having refreshed his IV bag.

Out I jogged back towards the fence, yelling, "Can someone come out, please!". No one. For the next couple of minutes I yelled and finally Gwyn came out along with two national nurses who were donned and at the front gate, waiting for their two walk-ins to be let inside. "Sorry to bother you but I'm going to need a body bag. Can you do that?"

Gwyn searched her brain. "I'll find a bag and you get Sally to the fence. There's a taxi waiting for the discharges to home."

With medicine, this situation of having to do five things at once is normal anywhere in the world medicine is practiced. In a short time, we'd accomplish discharges, admissions, a couple of patient shuffles, corpse removal and treatments. But unlike back home, here we'd be soaked to the bone and dipped in bleach before it was all over.

I went back in and updated Brett on the developments, to which he replied, "You can handle all that. Where's our body bag?"

"They're looking for one," I informed. "And here's the lab results on these two. We're supposed to take them over to confirmed."

Brett looked at the list and showed it to Dorine, then stuffed it into the ragbag he was carrying around with him. I asked Dorine to help me talk to Sally Kargbo to let her know she was being discharged to home and that there was a taxi to take her home. Dorine and I went to the foot of Sally's bed, where I asked Dorine to ask Sally if she was feeling OK. No headaches, hiccups, cough or weakness. Dorine scanned to see if her temperature was fine, which it was. Wordlessly, the young woman started gathering up her items and Dorine interrupted, speaking in Krio, breaking the news that anything brought into the hospital had to stay in the hospital and thrown away to be immolated in the burn pit. Sally looked at her cell phone and Dorine quietly shook her head, emphasizing with a soft 'no' that it, too, had to stay. Sally left her belongings, other than clothes she was wearing, and Dorine tossed them to the trash while I led her out, past the dead man on the floor. Sally just stared straight ahead, letting her eyes lead her out the door.

Outside, we walked across the courtyard to the shower, a faucet three feet up off the ground. I found soap, clean buckets and some rags that could be used as a towel. No matter how medical the situation was, a 54 year old man asking a 15 year old girl to get naked and shower is awkward at the least and creepy as anyone normal would think, but I coaxed her into it and she took it from there, giving me a chance to go back and check on the body bag and see if the admissions were coming along.

Sloughed over the blue tarp fence was the body bag, waiting for me. Two national nurses were questioning a mother with a 5 year old child, soliciting her for her symptoms and observing for signs of Ebola infection, quizzing if she or anyone in her family recently cared for someone who died where there was Ebola. She nodded or shook her head yes and no to the questions. I grabbed the bag and went into where the body was but Brett and Dorine weren't, then chased them down in the next building over, flashing the body bag.

Brett left his patient for Dorine to finish then he and I returned to the body. I could hear Brett's breathing, the sweat and moisture rattling about in his mask. We knelt to the floor and opened the bag, unfolding alongside and pushing it beneath the body. The bag unzipped and opened, Brett rolled the corpse onto the side, the backside completely soaked in diarrhea and probably vomit as well. Brett kept holding, then yelled, "Sprayer!" Out of a side room the sprayer appeared and saw what we were doing, knowing exactly what was needed of him. Pumping his lever several times, the sprayer waited for Brett to get out of the way and when he did he began dousing the inside of the bag then misted the body until visibly wet. Brett went back to his knees and again lifted the body up while I adjusted for length and width. The man was then left to fall into the bag and we tucked up the sides.

"Get the wrist band off," Brett instructed, which I did with a quick tug. "Take the information on the band and write it on top the bag." Brett zipped him up while I searched the mess of the table for a marker, found one and came back and copied the name, age, date of death onto the bag's topside and tied off the wrist band to the zipper tab.

"Now what?" I asked, worrying about Sally and the two admissions I had to take care of yet.

"Check on the admissions and get your discharge to the fence. I'm getting pretty warm." Brett's mask was soaked and you could hear it when he talked. Mine wasn't any better. Hustle time.

Back out at the shower, Sally was just finishing cleaning, naked. I nodded and turned my back to try to give her a sense of privacy and wait until she finished up, distracting myself by noticing that the scraggly weeds and plants were losing their green after a week without rain. Others were blooming with delicate small yellow flowers and some sort of morning glory type vine with a strong purple flower was peaking.

"OK," Sally spoke.

I turned. She had wrapped herself in one of the lafas put out for the purpose of drying and covering up for the walk to the gate at the fence. The sunshine sparkled in the drops of water in her hair, glimpses of rainbow shimmering. I tried to congratulate her on being able to go home but her grasp of English was about as good as my grasp of Temne and she continued with her flat affect.

The back door gate was strewn with discarded clothes, broken phones stomped on, sandals and shoes, buckets, towels and even a wallet or two. Two national nurses were on the other side waiting with fresh clothes for Sally while down the pathway a group of four was milling about. They noticed us at the gate, at which one of them yelled and they all ran down to the gate, one of them with tears streaming down her face. Family?

Sally broke out in a smile. The national nurses gave instructions for Sally to dress, which was my cue to turn my back as soon as I opened the gate for the clothes to be passed through by the nationals who would lay them over the stoop. I waited for permission to see her off and the nationals gave it. The last step was for Sally to step out of her sandals, place one foot outside into waiting new sandals, then the other. Free.

The four women and Sally wept quietly, not touching as instructed except for the elbow bump, then I watched as everyone walked up the drive to the road, glad she was going home in good health.

Racing back to the fence, I checked the admissions and they were ready. A mother and her 5 year old son were both running fevers with the mother looking the worst of the two. She was a walk-in who had come in by motorcycle taxi, a bad idea. A person could only hope she wasn't positive. Her physical, observable symptoms of red eyes and complaint of headaches, along with a fever of 102 working against her, she clutched her little boy, he with no shirt, saw me and buried his face in his mother's shoulder, certainly not enamored with the big white thing with only a pair of eyes staring out at him. I asked Gwyn about the other admission and she stated that they, out there somewhere, were still waiting for an ambulance to become available. Since there are only 5 in the district, it might be hours before one was ready. Mom quietly waited and I gathered up her admission bucket with toothpaste, brush, lafa, two 1.5 liter bottled waters and packets of Paracetamol and Valium to give to her when she was settled in. Both looked clean and denied diarrhea and vomiting, a definite plus.

We entered the final gate and walked over the hot gravel, up the concrete ramp to Suspect 5 where I heard other mothers and children were being housed. Inside, several mothers and kids were on the beds. A boy and a girl would go in and out to see the outside, then the mother would admonish them to come back in, not wanting them out of her sight. The others were trying to rest, their children lying with them close in on cholera beds, tenuously, where if anyone moved an inch one way, the other person would fall off. Some looked at the new arrivals while the others minded their own business, privacy a non-issue.

We found a corner and I motioned that this would be her bed space and set her bucket down, then explained supper would be around in a couple of hours. Also, that there was a faucet outside for cleaning up but that the water was not for drinking. Popping out 1000 mg of Paracetamol for the mother, and splitting one for the child, the mother took hers, then took the half pill and coaxed it into her fussy son. I pointed at the water bottles, "Wata", motioning she needed to drink, drink some more and keep drinking. She took the bottle and finished off half, then managed her son to take a cup. All good sign.

Back outside, Brett and Dorine had one of the transfers ready for confirmed waiting on the steps. Dragging out my name, Dorine instructed me, "Reeeck, go to admissions. Look if there is a wheelchair. Our patient inside is too weak."

Over at admissions, I found the wheelchair, all one of it. It was in the form of a wheelchair, but had been bleached down so many times that rust was overtaking the chrome and anything else metal, along with the black canvas fading out. Grabbing it and giving it a good shake to test its reliability and sturdiness, I concluded it would work. It had to; there was no other.

Inside Brett and Dorine stood by, waiting next to a thin, wet, and weak 50 or so year old patient. Positioning the chair sideways to the patient, Brett and Dorine lifted under his arms to get him into standing position, at which point he let loose with diarrhea, soaking his pants.

"Oh, shit," Brett carped.

Dorine, laughing, stated the obvious, "Ooooh, yes, it is."

While the pair held him up, I grabbed his trouser waistline and stripped down the pants, working each foot out, then grabbed a bottle of water and soaked one of our few rags, wiping off the offal as well as possible. Absorbability was not the strong suit of the material so it was more of smear at first until I resoaked the rags and went back over his fouled legs and glutes. Another rag to dry him and then a lafa wrap for where his pants used to be. Not a sound from the poor man.

Brett and Dorine dropped him in the chair and at the door we wheelied the front of the chair over the 6 inch high concrete door stoop, then lifted him over the rest of the way. Down the ramp and onto the gravel, large stones not conducive for narrow wheel chair wheels running on metal rims, the rubber off who knows how long ago, rattled the chair. Our patient slumped forward, stopped from falling out by Dorine who had anticipated this. Finally, onto the concrete walkway, the rolling was easier and we went through the gates.

Inside confirmed, most of the other workers were gone and in line for doffing. Dennis and Kelli were intent on a mother and her two babies. Mom was a mess but verbal, able to sit up enough to breast feed the two 8 month old twin girls who each eagerly latched on to a breast. A fresh IV was running on the mother and you could see on her arm the several failed IV starts covered with cotton and Band-Aid, her veins collapsed from dehydration and hard to find. Best to leave them alone and finish without interruption.

In the building over, about half the 20 beds were taken and we found a spot for our man and stood him up, sat him and swung him onto the bed. He rolled to his side away from us and Dorine encouraged him to take a drink but he refused. Brett, a step ahead, was rummaging the table for a 20 gauge needle, line and bag. I held the arm, while Brett hunted for a vein and decided on one. First poke and he had the red flash of success. While he taped down the site, struggling with the tape sticking to his gloves and trying to make sure the tape didn't pull a hole in his glove, it did exactly that. Breached.

"Damn," he said holding up the breached finger. "Not to worry; three pairs on." I finished lancing the bag and connecting the line to the new start and opened up the fluid stop wide, letting the saline solution pour through as fast as possible. Who would replace it in an hour after it was empty? Probably no one until morning. The poor fellow likely needed at least two, and three wouldn't hurt. The limits on our time and limits on the numbers available to do anything were still thin, leaving patients short of receiving a decent standard of care.

Tucked in and away, we stopped by Dennis and Kelli. Both were off the floor, having finished what they could do and were ready as anyone else to leave. The doffing station was clear, everyone else having finished and now out. While we waited turns as Dorine led off the process, four of us discussed what we did with the talk turning to the twins. The mother tested positive but both the twins were negative, so why were they in with her at all? It had been decided that her breast feeding very likely infected them and it was just a matter of time until the viral load increased enough to trip a positive PCR result, thus it made sense to let them be with her. However, 5 days had passed since admission to Confirmed and eight days since admission to Suspect. Mom was becoming more ill while the babies showed no signs or symptoms at all. Since Ebola takes on average about 7-12 days to make itself known, that was 15-20 days where Mom could have passed it on. It wasn't adding up and speculation was maybe there was a screwed up PCR on mom, and that it was malaria or something else and maybe she should be retested to confirm the initial results. We'd see.

After the bleach blast, it was good to be out of the PPE. Everyone was soaked to the bone. Back at the nurses' station, everyone was getting ready to leave and some had already gotten into shuttle service and went home. I was as ready as anyone else to go when a phone rang. It was my bag.

Digging it out of the backpack, it was Gwyn on the caller ID. "Rick, can you come over and help get our new admit in? The ambulance showed up."

'Dang it', I thought. "You mean suit back up and come in or come over there?"

"You can do it here or do it over there," Gwyn offered. "We have no nationals left who can go in."

"OK, I'll come over there and suit up when the patient is ready to be walked in."

Over I ran, going outside the fence, saying 'hello' to everyone I passed was something I found I'd do every time I travelled back and forth. J Edgar Hoover, the commanding police officer on duty, a name I gave him because I couldn't ever recall his proper given name, and a nickname he enjoyed after I explained who Hoover was in American history, flashed his big smile while he and his two cohorts listened to the BBC or some soccer game. The man couldn't hurt a fly but he had size and you can't teach size.

Inside, Gwyn was dressed in light gear, talking to the patient over the fence, writing down all the vitals and other information. She had me go back in to get the wristband and put together an admission bucket, which I did, then suited up. By the time I did all that, the patient, a young man of 25 or so, was ready and I placed his band, explained myself, what I'd do and who I was. He made a genuine attempt to be pleasant as I asked where he was from, how he was feeling and so on. Inside, Suspect 1, I decided it was best to give him his own space and put him around a corner that hid him from view of the others. He was a college graduate and had studied economics but had yet to get a visa to leave the country and look for better work. Soon, he thought he would have enough money as his family saved to achieve the goal. He was it. He was the family's Chosen One, the potential winning ticket for a better life. We weren't going be taking care of just one person but an entire family, maybe a clan. It was a moment like this where you knew this was more than trying to eradicate a disease and save a life; we were trying to save futures.

The whole process took 20 minutes and I walked through to doffing. No sprayers. The next five minutes were spent with me yelling out for a sprayer and finally Racin showed up to help me through the process, joking that I was making him work late.

Back at the nurses' station, only Dennis was waiting, telling me as I came through the door, "I thought I'd wait for you. How'd it go?"

I was happy to see him. All the drivers were gone. Instead of waiting, we decided to walk back the half-hour. I thought maybe I, we, some of us, would be more upset by the conditions but that was not the case, the reason being we all knew this was our beginning and that attempts would be made to improve what we needed to do. Some would work. As Dennis liked to say, it was a process. When we did need to change or add something, he'd quip, "Hey, how hard could it be." That of course means man has a tendency to underestimate and over promise. Like I said earlier, that's how the Donner Party became famous.

Up to Speed

What the Frontier Four saw in the month before we arrived was all the shortcomings that needed addressed. By confronting the same every day, they were able to prioritize what should be attacked first.

Francie, Brett, Kelli and Patti came into a place held together by string and staples and put themselves right into the thick of it along with the national nurses, an under supported, underfunded force of their own that was now possible thanks to the millions of dollars coming in from the developed world. For a fraction of the emergency response money, maybe a solid national health system could have been built that would have been more able to respond to the crisis. However, that's Monday morning quarterbacking on a hypothetical.

Walking to work was the morning norm for most of us, the weather as perfect as one could hope for, allowing us to learn what was sold where. Nothing was in great supply like you would find in stores back home. This was evident by the local woodworkers' tools that were 19th century by American standards, the same ones I'd seen hundreds of times collecting dust out it in a tool shed on my grandparent's farm in Wisconsin. A hand-powered drill to a kid is a toy but to an adult it is inefficient, a waste of labor when an electric drill did the same job in a fraction of the time. No grid, no 20th century.

Inside the ETU, keeping various items separated for easy finding was a problem. With everything—meds, tapes, needles—all in a pile on small plastic tables, a person had to sift and sort to find the one item needed to complete the task at hand. It was not in Dr. Galleo's nature to tolerate disarray. On one of the morning walks, he struck a deal for an order of two wooden boxes with a promise to order more if the first two were up to snuff. Looking at the carpenter's tools hanging on the stick walls, my first thought was it would take a week, maybe two, to put together what Galleo was ordering, all by hand gestures to indicate width, height and depth and compartments along with a hinged lid. The next morning, we had two pharmacy boxes and Galleo ordered eight more.

Some days, someone in the group would purchase toys for the kids or maybe pick up some spare lafas to hand out in the ETU to the patients. Francie hit the sweet spot for the kids by buying up all the soccer balls at one shop, 6 in all, and handing them out as presents for the surviving children at discharge. One was taken inside, but the kids were in no mood for games, as one might not be surprised to learn, so the soccer ball rested, unkicked, unnicked, unscraped and was about the best shape of anything inside the ETU. Galleo and Peterson bought a couple of radios to put inside so patients had something to listen to while they tried to erase the hours before they passed or went home. I can't hear a radio today without thinking of J Edgar at his perimeter post, listening to BBC news or soccer games, or recalling one of the healthier patients fiddling the dial to find music, then turning the volume up to the point where someone would have to go turn it off for the sake of harmony and peace inside the ETU.

The morning walks became progressively more dry, our clothes not sticking by the time we arrived. The yellow morning light was now competing with a red haze lightly saturating the cloudless days, a gritty dust you could taste on a breezier day as the northeasterly Harmattan winds came out of the Sahara desert along with cooler nights, necessitating a light wrap. The odor of burning grasses was now a constant as the locals undertook the annual practice of burning back the brush that grew up over the rainy season, clearing it from around the homes to keep the bugs and snakes at bay.

On this morning trek to work, fields of brush were torched and the fire starters simply walked away after ignition had been achieved. Soon, the fire raced through the dry brush, covering hundreds of feet in minutes and the grass hut that was someone's house across from the ETU, caught flame and was gone. Someone lived there. It was a place for someone to lay their head at night and get out of the rain, catch some shade, a place to eat and invite guests to, or just feel safe. Now it was a campfire, yellow-white smoke rolling off as flame made the palm leaves snap and pop. Where would the owner sleep tonight? What about his clothes, bedroll and maybe food? Did he have means to get by? Probably not; he was living in a grass hut. Every day it felt like there was something else to fix. Every day you had to remind yourself to stick to the things you could control.

The morning routine was to attend report in the admissions building and hear what Martin had to say about his morning round through the hospital, a laying on of the eyes to assess what had happened overnight, a roll call of the dead, alerts to who was likely next and some positive news for the end. Kelli and Dennis inquired about the mother and her 8 month old twins in Confirmed.

Over the past several days, mother would pull herself up onto one of the mattresses that were finally delivered one day by van, tied in a stack to the roof. Several more loads came in like this and made their way inside the ETU, resolving the issue of the high bed hazard for those who were in throes and not always aware of their position relative to the concrete floor. Situated with her back to one of the wall studs, her IV clogged off and IV fluid not keeping up with her hydration needs, she would pull the children to her breasts, brushing her nipple to their mouths to prompt them to latch. When she felt better, she would hum to the children as they suckled and she stroked their faces, resting her own cheek on their heads. Soon she was not humming but would still pull herself up, her back resting on the rough wall stud, soaked in her own sickly waste, and latch the twins who now worked hard for milk, enough so that their mouths hurt from the effort that they soon gave up, whimpering or crying out of hunger. White suits would come in twice a day and fill syringes with formula out of boxes that had been shipped from Freetown to quell the hunger. Everyone thought it was only soon before the twins would take ill and they would go to the cemetery to be placed next to mother. Mother did not consider her hastening mortality to be an excuse dismissing her maternal duties and, in her heart, it was the true purpose of her existence in the midst of her own ruin, surrounded by others feeling the fire of life cool hour by hour. During the night, the twins moved in closer to the prone body, curling up in the crux of her lap but not staying warm. In the morning the twins awoke and pawed at the breasts but mother did not sit up, their whimpering futile, so they waited for the white suits with the milk. The twins reacted to the abnormal coolness and curled in tighter to the complete stillness to feel what was left of mom's warmth before our fleshless white arms grabbed them for a feeding.

The white suits came in and the twins watched for the box and syringe, but the suits immediately left, prompting disappointment over their ignored hunger and so wailed in protest. The wailing worked and three white suits came back with two of them taking one each and moving across the room, placing them on an empty mattress to feed their eager stomachs. Two other white suits came in and sprayed mother where she lie, then unfolded the heavy vinyl, unzipped it, snatched the wrist band and rolled mother in, shutting her away for the carry down to the mortuary shelves where teams of 6 in Red Crescent/Red Cross trucks would arrive to pick up the day's endings.

"The mother with the twins in C-3, deceased," John matter of factly stated. The Major and Kelli merely nodded, having hoped for the best, knowing the worst can always happen here.

"But the twins are not sick," Kelli asserted. "We need another PCR on them. Something is happening ."

The Major chimed in, "No doubt something unusual is happening."

In a room of twenty medical professionals, 18 of them doubted the idea of these twins breast feeding off an Ebola infected mother not eventually becoming ill. We were witnessing the contagion. Impossible.

Gwyn was rifling her stack of papers, pulling up a lab schedule. "The twins had a PCR pulled two days ago. Results should be in later about noon."

Someone from the group asked, "How fast are labs getting turned around?"

"Two days," Gwyn delivered. "By the end of the week the Dutch hope to have the lab organized enough to get it to 24 hours. All they have to do is some staff training."

The lab was starting to hum so it made sense to divide the newly admitted patients waiting in Suspect units as wet or dry. Those not diarrheaing and vomiting would be kept apart from those who were, giving those who were negative/dry a safer environment to lower their infection risk. It would then be safer to discharge PCR negative suspect patients back into the community without added risk, to themselves or to those where they returned. There is no doubt certain dry patients were ensnared by the strict fever trigger for quarantine who were, in fact, not Ebola infected. However, their proximity to positive wet patients while they awaited test results sometimes ended with their becoming infected. These patients were discharged since they had no signs, symptoms and a negative test result but were walking time bombs released into the general public. The updating of admission assignment criteria was a step in the right direction.

The twins were dry even though they had been inside with their mother for nearly two full weeks plus when she fell ill nearly three weeks earlier, breastfeeding the entire time.

"We need those results and need to discharge them as soon as we can," Kelli stated.

"Wait for the labs and go from there," Doc Peterson offered in his Colorado drawl. "We still need to find family or someplace to take them—and that's a big 'if'. Can we say for certain these twins are not infected based on today's results anyways? By protocol, the 21 days starts this morning for them. Is it wise to let them out until then?"

Galleo returned, "Where do we put them? They're asymptomatic. No fever the whole time here. Yet, they've had the closest contact imaginable by breastfeeding, making it 100% they're likely infected. We keep them in Confirmed or back to Suspect? Home is not an option today, tomorrow or even next week."

"Listen," Kelli argued back, "those kids have been on an infected mom 3 weeks and not a single sign they're infected. I know it makes no sense but something is happening that these kids are not catching Ebola. I'm willing to bet right now that their PCR's come back negative." She emphatically added, any hint of a smile of accommodation gone, saying, "They're not sick and they're not going to get sick."

Even the Major had his doubts judging by the respectful skepticism on his face. Now it was more like 19 of 20 in the room believing it impossible. Everyone was in a position to guess but none of us were in a position to know.

As Americans, we are conditioned to the idea of patient autonomy and that we should always err on the side of the patient autonomy even to the point of self harm by omission. The only time this sacred right is violated is when the patient is no longer competent and even then we've created a system that begs persons, while competent, to give the rest of us direction and guidance, to appoint guardians. The twins had none of this. No family had made themselves known. The twins were on an endless sea, no shore in sight, and their rescue would belong to the first vessel to claim them. The mother never heard of a Living Will, Healthcare Power of Attorney or Assignment of Guardianship she could compose on behalf of her children. They had us. More specifically, they had Kelli and the Major since they were the two who had taken on the pediatric cases with great vigor and a budding success that looked promising.

My assignment was set so I left morning report meeting to round up the national nurse and sprayer Brett and I would be going in with. Outside the admissions' building door, resting workers were milling about, biding time until their next duty on the inside. In an 8-hour day, two 90-minute shifts inside leaves for plenty of free time, some of it spent preparing for the next trip in but still leaving as much as 3 hours to wile away. Of course, there are those who read this and think 'lazy', but that sort of ignorance is based on not understanding what heat can do to a body. Athletes, who workout in weather appropriate light gear, know that two 90 minute sessions a day in 90 degree heat is considered brutal and usually harmful. Late summer high school football programs encounter this tragedy when some knucklehead coach tries to toughen his players up by having them perform maximum workouts in shoulder pads and helmet. Some poor kid drops, ending up going for an ambulance ride thanks to heat stroke or heat exhaustion. Many workers had been working for weeks without a day off, a mental grind magnifying the physical challenges.

As I walked down the perimeter fence line, the usual cadre of folks was present and the same cadre continued to shout out as I walked. By doing so, an obligation was set down that I felt I needed to take up and respond with small chit chat. J Edgar snoozed outside his guard house, keeping one eye open as usual, then rose off his bench to greet me.

"Mr. Rick, good morning," J Edgar greeted in his typical broad smile.

"You have people looking for you. Come." He led me back towards the admission building and pointed to the Tree of Life, a memorial space out in front with branches covered in bows and ribbon placed by discharged survivors. J Edgar pointed at two men sitting on the concrete edge of the bowl that surrounded the tree, saying, "They want to talk to someone about a patient who is inside. Can you help them?"

For me? Who would want to talk to me about anything. I could never remember anyone's name once I left the hot zone, making giving report a real hit and miss affair for anyone who followed when I tried to pass on information, instead relying on their location in the building along with age, sex and who they might be near.

The two men, one maybe 50 and the other about 35, stood up as I approached. I stopped in front of them and introduced myself. "Hello. I'm Rick, one of the nurses here. The officer said you wanted to speak with someone?"

The older gentleman smiled and with a dignity that exuded status, spoke respectfully, "I am Muhammad Sesay and this is my brother, Musa Sesay. We are hoping for news of my son, Osman Sesay. Can you tell us anything?"

It was the colorful hat and how Muhammad wrapped himself that conveyed to me he was a man rarely seen in informal clothes. His diction was perfect and deliberately precise, possibly revealing he often dealt with people of position where English was the preferred language. Muhammad's brother, stoic, was dressed more typically in day to day wear of short sleeved shirt and jeans.

I was drawing a blank. Sesay was a common name. Osman meant nothing. I racked my head and apologized, "I'm sorry, I can't place the person. Can you tell me when he came here?"

"One week ago," Muhammad pronounced. "We've traveled since early this morning a distance of 80 kilometers. Please let this not be a waste of time."

Muhammad's pleading was more a statement that I not dismiss him, which I would not. "Let's go inside here," I said, pointing the admissions building. "There is a list of names I can go through and that might help me locate who is taking care of your son."

Inside, the morning report had broken up and Gwyn was handling her phone like a weapon, slicing the red tape away to get things done. The bandage on her wrist was now more of a sweatband, her wound probably healed well enough, but now she was a master of the admissions' universe and no one wanted to blow that up, including her, thankfully.

"Gwyn," I interrupted, "is there an Osman Sesay on the board here somewhere you recall.   These two gentlemen are looking for information."

We both went down the four boards on the walls, hunting for an Osman. "How old?" Gwyn inquired.

"25 years," Muhammad replied.

Gwyn spotted the name and pulled the tag off the one of the two confirmed boards, reading it aloud. "Osman Sesay. 25. Admitted on the 6th." She handed it to me and the four of us crowded in to read all the information contained in black and red marker.

I looked up at the two men, who were eager for news. "I do know your son. I've helped take care of him and I admitted him." It was his red dress sweater and white dress shirt that I remembered, then recalled the mnemonic I was using on him: Osman equaled Osmond, like Donny Osmond the singer and conservatively dressed like Donny Osmond. I thought Osman would fit right in Salt Lake City.

"Will he be coming home?" Muhammad quietly asked.

"I don't know, sir. I just don't know," I shook my head, continuing, "Osman tested positive three days ago for Ebola," I said, holding the board note so it could be read. "He isn't feeling well but he does get up to walk and I've seen him cleaning himself, both good signs."

Muhammad nodded, taking it in, asking, "What is being done for him?"

In detail, I explained how we were encouraging him to drink and eat and he was getting IV fluids to battle his dehydration. Additionally, our protocol was now treating patients with antibiotics like Cipro, Flagyl and erythromycin to battle back any opportunistic secondary infections that too often settled on the Ebola positive patients. At best, it would be probably 4 or 5 days before we'd know if he was out of the woods. I explained that since our group's arrival two weeks earlier, more patients were surviving and leaving for home, the 90% mortality rate now at about 50%, a flip of the coin fighting chance rather than a near mathematical certainty of death. Osman's father and uncle took this in, listening intently, nodding they understood.

After a pause, Muhammad Sesay spoke. "Osman has a student visa for Great Britain. He is to go to King's College for advanced studies in economics, a scholarship arranged by the Sierra Leone government."

The import of this information was not lost on me. In this country, the government doing something of this nature was a considerable investment, literally a winning ticket. I made an offer. "I am going inside in the next hour. In about two hours, at 11 o'clock, if he is strong enough to walk I can bring him to the fence in back and you can see and speak with him, providing Osman agrees to this. Would you like me to do that?"

The uncle, quiet, brightened, "Absolutely. I wish to see my nephew." Muhammad shook his head in consent.

After pointing out where I would bring Osman to and reiterating the time, the two took a seat on the ground in the shade of a tree on the near outside the fence. Reaching into my school bag for the water bottle, I offered it to them to keep and they thanked me as they settled in for the wait.

I jogged back to the nurse's station, connected with Brett and rounded up Dorine and a sprayer. Others were already donning and we had yet to gather up any of our supplies though there were plenty of water bottles ready to go, the ORS mixed in. Rummaging through the nurses' station drawers, we bagged antibiotics, needles, IV fluids, tabs of tape, rags and IV line.

Being the last in, we went straight to our assigned buildings, Confirmed 3 and 4, and began administering treatments as dictated by the patient bedside charts that finally came through and were now on the end of every bed. This took the guesswork out of who got what when, if they had received it, and charting their decline or improvement by way of signs and symptoms. This mattered in that patient's were now on scheduled pharmaceutical regimens to maximize the effectiveness of the available drugs to administer and was especially important with Artemisinin, a malaria medication, something more than a few Ebola patients were simultaneously battling alongside Ebola. Most importantly, it knocked down the need to try to memorize who was who and what was the treatment regimen. By taking in commonly used items, we carried our own inventory and had it immediately available. One would think our hospital would have been cheered for these advances but certain powerful and respected groups considered it a waste of effort, so much so that one organization published a New York Times piece going so far as to argue that IV fluids were not needed for any Ebola patient who could drink even a little water on their own. It was painfully obvious that the designation of PO positive, meaning able to take fluids by mouth without assistance, was meaningless. Many patients could drink and get the water bottle to their lips of their own power, but the problem was that too many were too nauseas or weak to drink the 5 to 6 liters replacement fluids a day they were losing due to diarrhea and vomiting. It is not PO positive if a patient is drinking a third of a liter all day and losing 20 times that amount. Technically, yes, they are PO positive but the designation under such circumstances was absurd, leading some practitioners to avoid IV starts by claiming that the patient was able to drink on their own when it was transparent they were not able to stay hydrated. The revised protocol was the reason patient mortality dropped from 90% to 50%. Yet, some argued against the obvious. This was disappointing and worrisome as some of them held power and could upend it all if they pushed the right buttons.

Brett and Dorine checked IV's and rehung bags while I checked the charts to see what meds the patient needed. Dorine asked the questions of the patients regarding headache, nausea, fatigue, hiccups, etc. and I would check off 'Y' or 'N', write in the scanned temperature and read out loud the medication regimen they were on and what should be given how. We hung bags of antibiotics on nails in the wall studs, a bright step up in infrastructure from a week ago. One of us would squeeze the bag to run the 250 ml in as a bolus dose, followed by a liter of normal saline, trying to cover as many patients possible in two hours. Some medications that came in with us were injectables for the patients, meaning it was safer to reconstitute in the safety of the nurses' station since several needle changes were involved in the mixing process. The risk of a stray needle poke and a million dollar plane ride home was greatly reduced by doing medication prep outside the red zone where things were less chaotic and more relaxed.

We maneuvered around full buckets of waste, food litter, soiled lafas and discarded clothing. Small talk was minimal since our patient load was increased, Maforki having become the major Ebola treatment hub for the Port Loko district with over 80 beds. In the last week, on any given day, 50 or more patients were present and the numbers continued to climb. We hustled through until I guessed it was 11 o'clock then I let Dorine and Brett in on Osman and his family visit. Dorine tracked him down in a corner, sitting on the side of the bed waiting for us. She began his assessment, checking off the boxes.

"Osman Sesay?" Brett asked.

Osman nodded, his eyes bloodshot.

"Osman, pull down your pants. We're giving you an antibiotic shot today to save time." Brett moved in with the syringe as Osman struggled with the waistband of his pants, eventually getting them down enough to expose his left gluteus. Brett took quick aim and Osman grimaced quietly. Meanwhile, I had a hung a fresh liter and was running it wide open, squeezing it to run it faster and finish out the liter so I could hang another.

"Osman," I said as I crushed his bag, "you have family here who want to see you. It's your father and uncle."

Osman stared back at me. "Do they have news?"

Osman had been moving slowly, obviously weak and preferring to simply rest on his cot and quietly fight, letting us do what we needed with neither approval nor objection.

"News? Are you expecting some news?"

"I'm waiting to see if I go to university in England. I am supposed to know this month if my visa and application have been approved."

He didn't know. "They're waiting at the fence," I said. "Do you think you can walk?"

Osman pulled himself up with a helping hand into sitting position, then reached for his still meticulously clean red sweater. His liter of IV fluid was nearly done and Dorine disconnected the line, helping Osman dress, wiping his face and mouth clean. Standing, he wobbled. He wasn't walking to the fence. Brett went outside and came back in with our jalopy of a wheelchair and sat Osman. Brett and Dorine offered to finish the several patients if I felt I could handle wheeling Osman over to the fence. I was more than happy to take a stroll out in the yard and away from the misery inside the unit.

Beneath the shade of the trees just outside the fence, Osman's visitors occupied themselves on their phones. On hearing the wheelchair rattling towards them, Osman and me navigating the rough stones and brush, the two snapped their phones shut and grasped the wire fence, their fingers looping over the wire. Giving the chair one last hard push, I let it settle two feet away, enough that if Osman were too reach out he would not be able to touch. Both elder men looked down at what was left of their noble son and nephew, frowns of dismay and disbelieving sadness painting their countenances. Osman's once muscular frame was diminished, his radiant complexion flat and blue tinged and his skin folding and tenting in places usually seen on the elderly.

"Osman?" Muhammad asked, knowing it certainly was.

Osman lifted his head, shaking and shivering slightly from the weakness that consumed him, and simply looked, expressionless, letting the obvious tell his tale.

I retreated to about 15 yards away, sitting myself on the discharge shower concrete bench to allow privacy.

Muhammad and Musa, the uncle, spoke slowly and softly, exchanging looks and gestures with one another and repeating back to Osman what they decided to ask. Osman sat, looking at the ground, speaking in short barely audible answers. There was a pause and silence before Muhammad pulled out a manila envelope, retrieving a letter he held up to the fence, then rolled it and pushed it through, looking at me to come and retrieve the writing as Osman could not reach it. I got up and grabbed the letter and offered it to Osman, who lifted his arm to accept but his hand missed, his fine motor control off, and the letter fumbled to the gravel as we missed the handoff. Picking it back up, I again offered it when Muhammad decided to paraphrase the letter as I held the letter open in front of Osman's face.

"Osman Sesay," Muhammad Sesay announced, "you have achieved. It is the acceptance of your scholarship application and letter of national support." Muhammad smiled. Musa looked at the ground then up and out to the distant forests. Osman managed a slight smile and to say, "Good," and nothing else, looking back to the ground.

From a distance, I heard Dorine's raised voice, "Reeeck! It has been long enough inside! You must go!" Muhammad and Musa understood and gave me a wave they were finished, with both men speaking Temne to Osman in what as best I could decipher was a farewell of best wishes. The two men watched as I wrestled the wheelchair around in the gravel and back across the courtyard, weaving through the sticks and brush until I was back on the concrete pathway in front of Confirmed.

"Turn me," Osman ordered. I swing the wheelchair 180 degrees so he could see his relatives as they left. Muhammad was on a knee with Musa's palms on Muhammad's shoulder as Muhammad pulled himself up, then both men turned and walked down the drive toward the exit to the road out front, disappearing beyond the tarped fence. Osman took his letter, crumpled it and threw it on the ground, exclaiming, "There was no need for me to know."

With an assist, Osman stood up and sat himself on his bed. In unison, we took his legs and swung them until he was full on the bed deck. I hung another liter of IV fluid and found a clean lafa to cover him in hopes of ameliorating the jagged edge of the chill from his cutting fever. He agreed to 10 mg of diazepam to help him rest, putting the yellow pills into his mouth, coaxing small sips of water over his lips and tongue to wash the medicine towards his mind.

Patients called out as I left, this round over. They'd have to wait until afternoon. My breathing was audible and wet, each breath bubbling with snot, tobacco juice and general perspiration as a whiff of claustrophobia skimmed me until I shewed it away with a thought of it being a protective cocoon that gave me the super power of walking into, through, and away from deadly disease. As I crossed onto the porch, the crumbled letter rubbed under my boot. I picked it up, unrumpled it, refolded it and walked back in to put it on Osman's pile beneath his bed. He might want that someday.

Doffing was quick work without a line. After washing, I ducked back down to the nurses' station for some lunch, a spicy meat sauce over white rice and a fortified bottle of water with a handful of salt to ward off cramps that would haunt me at night if I didn't replenish.

Staff milled about, coming in and out, exchanging what went on inside and their assessments of who had the best chances and who didn't. Over the other side of the walkway, sprayers and cleaners, all men, were lined up for their payday, going in and out of the Maforki office as their turn came. For payday, some were not too happy judging by the scowls on their faces.

The Major and Kelli came inside and turned a fan on themselves after clearing a spot on the chairs, peeling open their lunches.

"Did you get the PCR results on the twins?" I asked.

Kelli looked up, smiling, "Negative."

"Let's try and not get ahead of ourselves," Dennis cautioned.

Francie, puttering at the desk, turned, and in her direct fashion, asked, "Why not?" Continuing in her French heavy accent, saying, "How long do they have to keep testing negative? They've been on the mom the three or four weeks since she became infected." Waving her hand, "And nothing. They should go home today. This place is not healthy for them."

Dennis replied in the neutral, saying, "Technically, we're supposed to wait 21 days since last exposure. Will anyone---does anyone---have the capacity to do that outside of us? As far as I know, I don't think so."

Kelli dug in, saying, "If we wait for 21 days from last exposure, they'll never get out of here until the last patient leaves. It could be months, a year. Every day is a new exposure. I say we have Musa and Gwyn call Catholic services for placement. There's no known family."

"I agree," Francie punctuated. "Negative is negative. We wash and

81

disinfect them as best we can. Two people go in. One goes into get dirty and do the first shower. The second person, clean, not having touched a thing, wraps the kids and walks them to the fence. Unwrap them and place the kids on a clean wrap. Done. No Ebola out the fence."

Musa, a man I never met, walked by, Kelli yelling him down, "Musa. Come here please."

Musa turned and came up the walkway. His size was notable, looking like he might have been a football lineman. When the crisis hit, Musa figured he owed his homeland and returned to offer his help after being naturalized into the United States 23 years earlier and making a home in Pittsburgh. All this I found out later. His English was no different from other Midwesterner's, colloquialisms and all, leaving me to believe, incorrectly, that Musa was born and raised in the Midwest. Back in America, Musa was a state social worker for at-risk youth.

Kelli offered Musa the story of the twins and explained their current condition and predicament. The rest of the conversation kept arriving at inconclusive and what protocol demanded and advised, leaving a frustrating Catch-22, a circle of logic where each question yielded more questions when an answer was needed. The talking ended when Musa promised to probe the predicament and start making phone calls to see if there was a chain of command that guided a decision or if Maforki would be completely winging it.

For now, the twins were in a box by themselves, separated by four cardboard sides from the rest of the patients, like it is done with puppies or kittens. The few times I attended the pediatric patients in confirmed, I noticed the last names on the wrist bands did not always match with mom's, meaning children who came in alone or lost their parent while inside, were gathered in and looked out for by surviving mothers. There were no objections from children or mothers. With the natural order of things disrupted, maternal instinct rewove the rented fabric of family into blankets of protection.

Debate rolled on up the chain of command and the twins' predicament was soon to be a precedent in deciding how children would be separated from parents when test results were negative for one and positive for the other considering the natural physical closeness infants and toddlers had with their mothers. The normal acts of love---kissing, grooming, caressing—were ultra high-risk modes of transmission of Ebola from mother to child. The question of breastfeeding babies was a no brainer: of course they would be infected. There is nothing magical about breast milk killing the virus or preventing transmission to a child. Yet, here were two perfectly healthy breastfeeding twins who for three weeks drank the breast milk of their infected mom who succumbed. Everything known about Ebola was blowing up in our faces.

The twins' negative results created a crisis that jumped the fence and rolled out into the wider medical community of how to handle such a unique situation. First, was it even possible Musa could raise an agency to agree to take these children and, if they were willing, would they be able to follow a protocol of no physical contact using PPE and disinfecting routines. Musa worked his phone. Gwyn, in addition to her overwhelming duties keeping patients coming and going from all over the district in smooth form, jumped in, going so far as to put a well connected national on notice of the events in case some political muscle would be needed to get the ball in the net.

The ethics became twisted since individual patient autonomy was trumped by national concern, the rights of the patient muted. Starting there, the debates amongst the various clinicians, managers and pols emphasized the known: people who had close, hands on contact with Ebola positive victims, especially the recently deceased and those close to passing, were high risk and needed to be treated and cared for as if they were positive, requiring quarantine under a 21 day observation period. This made sense to everyone.

Then there was the hard reality: two 8 month children had as close of contact as humanly possible, including consuming fluids, from an infected mother for a period of three weeks and still tested negative. Would keeping them in Confirmed increase their risk of infection from casual contact via other patients and the healthcare workers who would be handling, cleaning and feeding the children? Was their uninfected status due to some sort of viral quirk that rendered Ebola vulnerable to antibodies contained in breast milk, or was it a quirk of the twins' immunity that rendered the mother's particular strain of Ebola impotent within them?

The outside possibility was that the mother died of something other than Ebola, that she had been misdiagnosed completely. The likelihood of a false positive was remote, though in medicine nothing is impossible and for those that consider all possibilities as healthy skepticism, it can also sometimes paralyze the decision process, wasting precious time pondering instead of treating.

The Port Loko Catholic Charities orphanage made Musa's day and agreed to consider taking in the twins based on the condition their staff would have access to medical expertise, a doable item.

Eventually, the reasons that prevailed were it would be harmful to continue to keep the twins within the hospital and risk their becoming infected, and that a 21 day quarantine in a safer more appropriate environment would suffice using standard precautions of PPE and disinfectant.

Prevailing in this case meant those closest to the twins, the Maforki staff on sight, were pulling the levers of power to arrange the outcome. Up and down the lines of hierarchy that stretched out over the globe involving government and nongovernment organizations, opinions differed and the troubling answer reaching our ears was bureaucratese, words emphasizing caution more out of a fear of being wrong than achieving a conclusion. Risk aversion is natural. However, healthy skepticism can degenerate into indecisiveness where higher powers become prone to self-preservation, thus mastering the art of being non-committal while peddling it as thoughtful consideration, a typical day's work. Waiting for their minds to be made up was no benefit to the situation.

By the end of the day, a van arrived to ferry away the twins, a national nurse accompanying the two children along with two nuns who would be trained how to monitor the children and protect themselves. The undercurrent of doubt, our fear, was we were sending out two possibly infected children into an orphanage and, despite the safeguards, it would result in a disaster. It was at this moment as a collective community our faith was as strong as anyone's serving a church that has stood for 2,000 years. Reason and rational rest on stones of fact; faith is what allows us to act and live with the results. I hoped that for 21 days it would be out of sight, out of mind and the twins would go on to be embraced by those outside the fence.

By force of personality, Kelli achieved the compassionate outcome while being cognizant of the risks, correctly surmising that non medical people, like nuns, could be capably instructed to watch over the twins. After all, they were hardly inexperienced with sickness and illness within the walls of their mission and often time served as the local medical professionals, having served for years many times under the tutelage of other caregivers. Like the Major said, "How hard could it be?"

Could You Repeat That, Please

When we arrived at 8 a.m., another bus would unload a pile of medical professionals of doctors and nurses who would go through the gates, then for the rest of the day, become invisible unless you accidentally met one using the rest room down the walkway. There were many other-nationals, as I self referenced them, ranging from the Dutch who set up the labs, to the British who provided communications and logistical support, to the Irish who built outlying clinics and treatment facilities in more rural areas. The only time I ever came across them was to drive past their respective bleach white tent compounds of luxury with high speed internet, holiday parties that included feasts of 6 course dinners of lobster, steaks, wine and champagne, hot showers, all day electricity and a park like atmosphere where one could lounge under beautiful palms on manicured grounds. But our Ghetto had cute lizards and the occasional bop in the head from a sonar glitched bat along with a dog who scratched too much for his own good. What's Africa without the wildlife. No one visited us. Everyone wanted to hang at places not ours. The people on the bus who arrived every morning kept their own company. However, this morning they followed us down the front path to the admissions building for morning report.

Outside the east front gate, a small Cuban flag hung flat. The Cubans had predated our arrival and were involved in much of the hands on treatments until one of their comrades fell ill from Ebola, upsetting the apple cart back in Havana, which then ordered them to cease until safety protocols were reviewed and revised. They were out of the action for weeks, long enough that they were essentially absent except for staying holed up in their own nurses' station behind ours. If quiet is what makes a good neighbor, they were the best.

Our little morning report was comfortable inside but the arrival of 15 more bodies changed the dynamic . Where one once could get a seat to listen and write, now you resigned yourself to stand or scootch onto a corner of desk, peering through gaps of heads and shoulders at the speaker giving morning report.   What we instead received in that morning report was a grand announcement of bilateral international relations being instituted at Maforki ETU. The Cubans had gotten past that whole Bay of Pigs thing and agreed to team up with the capitalist-imperialists who had cast a jaundiced eye on the godless island communists for over 60 years. The embargo on them accomplished exactly zero but kept US commie haters happy, able to plausibly brag up to their respective voters about their commie hating credentials.

Adam and I grabbed a corner of the room to hear out the announcement. Adam had finally arrived but not before being detoured into Liberia for a week where the outbreak was now under excellent control. The need for his help was no longer viable or sensible. He was needed here as our case loads climbed. Today was his first day at the ETU.

"What's up?" he asked.

"It looks like the Cubans are going to be working inside," I guessed. "Adam," I confided my ignorance, asking, "you speak any Spanish?"

"Some," he nodded. "But I think Cuban Spanish is sort of different than Mexican Spanish. Anyways, I know a little."

"Probably commie Spanish," I joked.

The Cuban delegation spokesperson, Enrique, came forward and launched into his welcome speech, summarizing the history of the Cuban role in the Ebola response and then showering praise on the unity of Cubans and Americans with words like 'historic' and 'epic' and many, many other words I couldn't understand due to his thick accent and my tin ear. As Enrique spoke, he would punch the air with his arms, spread them wide and smile like a man who had achieved a long sought dream. If meeting Adam and me were it, I think the shine might come off pretty quick, thanks to my lead ear for Cuban accented English and

Adam's bartender Spanish. After many minutes more, Enrique wound up his Ode on International Co-operation by going about the room and bumping elbows, posing for as many pictures as he spoke in seconds, slapping and bumping the Major and just about anyone else he could get himself near enough. In the corner, I was good, safe from the Hug Monster.

"How's this going to work out," I whispered to Adam. "I can't speak Cuban. I'm not so sure learning US English has been on their high priority list the last 50 years. They probably speak fluent Russian."

Adam sighed, thin smile, and shook his head, "Don't worry. I'm pretty sure they'll keep us in teams based on nationality."

Enrique, done with his pictures, resumed the front of the room. "Today, us, the Cubans, will be going on a tour of the hospital." He clapped his hands hard and shook his arms for emphasis, adding, "We work in 6 hour shifts with one for the morning rounds and a new shift for the evening round. Tomorrow, we go in as Cuban, American and Sierra Leonean. Each team with each of us different," Enrique smiled in triumph, jabbing a finger in the air.

No cheers went up and it was quietly accepted that the new teams would happen going forward as much was feasible numbers wise. Up until this moment, language was a non-issue with all the Sierra Leonean nurses having been formally schooled in English, making communication issues a moot point and allowing for stumble free planning and obtaining vital patient information by way of their Krio and Temne language skills regards the patients, and then skillfully translated back into English for thuds like me.

I had to say something to somebody. "What the Sam Hill is he talking about?"

Adam stared at me, then replied, "He said, 'Tomorrow we're going in as mixed teams of Cubans, Americans and...'"

"I know that!" I interrupted. "This is not, I repeat, not a good idea to mix us together unless we can know we're going to be able to comprehend one another. Man, this could really suck." I was not anticipating good results.

Adam tried to put a good face on it all, "Hey, hard could it be?" Laughing it off as a minor annoyance at worst, which for him might well be since he spoke at least some Spanish, an idea I was quickly disabused of when we mingled after The Speech with our new colleagues. It became clear that any Spanish anyone in our group knew was generally marginal. The one redeeming feature was that some of the Cubans were acceptable with their English but they were at best 5, maybe 6, English speakers, meaning that the numbers game meant language issues. Throw in the local national nurses whose ears were as attuned to Cuban accented English as mine, and it was not a net plus.

The best way to act on patient assignments was to hand over a portion to the Cuban delegation, eliminating the language issues and the stress that would come from trying to work around these issues. However, I kept the thought fairly private and to myself. I really just wanted to swear; the obvious wasn't being grasped. Each round in the hot zone had physical limits. Cooler days were on us and likely the best days of the year we were going to have, giving us as much as two hours each round wrapped in full gear. The Cubans were limited to 1 hour and one round on their 6 hour shifts. The Cubans available for 10 a.m. rounds would not be available for the 2 p.m. round, meaning that whoever was paired up with them would be on a new learning curve every afternoon.

In the American hospital system, any float nurses or doctors filling in for the regular staff will tell you that the challenge is learning the ins and outs of your patient, their history, predilections, weaknesses, strengths, medication regimen and status of progression or regression. Knowing the patient on a personal and medical level, seeing the Big Picture, allows the nurse or doctor to anticipate problems and solve them before they are big problems, to work more efficiently and accurately. As important, you learn who the other treating clinicians are and become familiar with their habits to craft a more seamless delivery of care. As a float nurse myself for years, the stress of that job was the constant relearning of an entirely new patient assignment daily, some days every four hours if the shift was split between two or three departments. It's no accident that long-term care nurses and home nurses, jobs where patient turnover is quite low by hospital standards, know far more about their patients than the average hospital floor nurse, allowing for a higher quality of care in general.

Do people in medicine know this? That a constant reassignment of personnel contributes to poorer patient outcomes, higher caregiver stress and higher rates of error? Yes, but it is often ignored for reasons of hubris, meaning that since we all survived rigorous academic and clinical programs it is assumed we should be able to manage constant change with equal expertise on every patient as those who carry more consistent assignments. Nothing could be more damaging, infuriating and reckless.

A few years back, I read a book by a popular surgeon who enjoyed documenting the bureaucracy of medicine as he experienced it. One of his stories was how a new surgical approach and technique for a common type of GI surgery was being instituted, a radical departure from the old method, by his description, that would take time to learn and master. One surgeon insisted on multiple surgeries with the same team of operating room personnel for two weeks while the other surgeons continued to accept surgeries as assigned under the old random system, leaving those in the old system trying to learn the new techniques with maybe only one or two surgeries weekly, each surgery with different team members. The surgeon who pushed for multiple weekly surgeries with the same team mastered the new surgical techniques far more rapidly than his peers, so much so that his team members were taken from him to tutor the surgeons who were receiving only one or two opportunities a week to learn the new methods. Repetition of practice creates skill. I taught myself to be a competent IV start nurse not by doing one or two sticks a week but by asking if I could do as many as possible for a couple of weeks, a teaching lesson that paid great dividends in skill, confidence and knowledge.

Part of the problem is the bumper sticker medical education bromide of 'see one, do one, teach one'. There is no job skill in any profession I know of where seeing something done once qualifies a person as competent then to teach it. Learning a task is best done in as high as a quantity possible in as short a period of time as possible for best comprehension and mastery. The entire apprentice, journeyman and master system is predicated on time and frequency of practice which yields a mastery of skill.

Starting the next day, every round would be international staff with built in communication hurdles. The group as a whole put the best face on all of this as a noble and grand international effort. This would deliver better care while simultaneously overcoming historical and political divisions of the past century between two Cold War rivals. In truth, the Cuban doctors and nurses were skilled clinicians that would be of great help inside the hot zone. I just wasn't sure if pairing one or two up with me, a non Spanish speaking gringo, would be the best utility of their talents or mine. I've been wrong before and was probably overreacting, as Adam said. After all, how hard could it really be?

Patient census was running higher. The daily DERC reports (District Emergency Response Census) showed a steady upward climb of new cases with the majority being shunted to Maforki ETU, and it was obvious in the all the new names on the board every morning. On some days poor Gwyn was getting clobbered with 12, 14, 16 admissions. This meant a steady stream of ambulances, phone calls and clawing out of information over the phone from heavily accented speakers where instructions had to be repeated and rephrased two and three times to ascertain information.

One of us would be assigned either to the morning or afternoon to help admission team with the arrival of new patients, retrieve them from the ambulance, help assess their medical status, wrist band them and take them inside to their bed in Suspect until lab results returned to move them to Confirmed or discharge them to home.

Complicating the new cases and the extra work they were bringing with them, was the additional discharge work, a blessing made possible by the new staff and the more aggressive and comprehensive treatment protocols that were now paying off in a survivor rate ticking up to 60%. This was the singular most gratifying development I had ever been involved with in my life.

I was on the afternoon admission and discharge team for the first time, sparing me the sweatbox of PPE for the afternoon. Sitting inside the admissions building, it made my head spin to watch Gwyn and her national team make phone call after phone call, organizing the parade of patients in and out of the hospital, writing up new board tags, putting the lab numbers and results to the names on the board and deciding who would go where and when.

On the bench next to me, assigned the same duty, was Dr. Jabari Haja, a former Sierra Leonean like Musa, who now lived in the United States and had more degrees than I had fingers and toes. Jabari worked as a professor of pharmacology at a big city Ohio university and, like Musa, returned to his native country to lend what help he could to his former compatriots. His laugh and smile chased away any apprehension I had about the new assignment, leaving me confident in the knowledge he would walk me through any questions or problems as they came up. It helped immensely he was fluent in Krio and Temne to facilitate speaking with the patients who knew little or no English, which was now becoming more of an issue as more of the patients were coming from outside the Port Loko area from the more rural parts of the country where education, in general, was less available. Then Gwyn called us outside.

"Rick and Jabari, there's a truck outside with supplies. Can you help out?" Gwyn asked.

"Oh, no, I think my back is acting up but Rick isn't busy." Jabari then broke out in his ever constant laughter. "Of course."

So my partner turns out to be a higher grade of smart ass who finds the humor in the darkest of places. I guess this will be a ton easier than doing hot zone rounds.

Outside, the panel truck is packed with mattresses, donated clothes and buckets for the hot zone. We swarmed the truck and stacked items off to the side to take in as needed later. After the first part of the truck was unloaded, 80 pound blue bags of rice were tossed towards us to carry into the inside storeroom, the back of the truck high enough that one bag could be slid onto a shoulder for the 50 foot trip through three doors to the storeroom. With six of us, quick work was made of the errand, though my back was objecting after the 7th or 8th trip but none the worse for wear.

Job accomplished, Jabari found the joke in it all, remarking, "Excellent work. What would normally take two or three men we did with nine."

My expectation of a non-sweat afternoon was in ruins, my scrubs soaked. Then Gwyn collared us again for our assigned tasks.

"We have two admissions and one discharge. Can I get you fellows to walk them?" Gwyn asked, more out of being polite.

"What do I do?" I asked.

"Don all your gear like you normally would," Jabari counseled, adding, "but in your case put on two of everything." Then he walked me back to the donning room to help me dig out the gear, laughing at his joke.

Josephine, a smartly dressed national whose job it was to watch the store room and keep track of its contents, helped sort us out by finding gloves that fit, wrapping us in our aprons and writing 'Admissions' in big red letters on us, allowing us to jump to the front of the line at the doffing station so we could return, be ready and go should any other patients need to be brought in or moved. "Don't be slow. It is going to get busy."

"Not for me," Jabari pronounced, "but it will for Rick. I'm going home."

"Dressed like that? Right," I ribbed back.

"Yes, damn it, 5 o'clock is 5 o'clock," Jabari mockingly asserted, then laughed so hard Josephine stepped back, shaking her head, acting as if this was too unprofessional even for her laid-back tastes.

Outside, under the newly built admissions area Francie willed into existence, there was cover from the elements and some privacy. An ambulance had backed inside. Two national nurses were offering their hands to help both men hop down off the back bumper. The sprayer immediately misted the nurses, then the nurses directed the pair to take a place in the available plastic chairs. Jabari and I looked on as the nurses took temperatures, examined mouths, eyes, and general overall condition, questioning the pair about recent possible Ebola contacts, filling in the boxes on the admission sheet regarding signs and symptoms. Finally, both were given IV's. This was the new protocol for all new admits. The new arrivals were capable of traveling under their own power.

Gwyn came out and gave Jabari a pair of wristbands to hand to the nurses. Josephine put together a bucket for each with toothpaste, toothbrush, bottled water, leftover lunch tins, lafa and sandals. The national nurses administered Paracetamol to each patient for their fevers and pain, something the patients reluctantly participated in, overwhelmed by where they had arrived. Their eyes scanned the surroundings, trying to comprehend the situation in which they now found themselves. One of the nurses produced two lab vials, one for each patient. She inserted the butterfly needle into the antecubital cephalic vein until dark red blood filled each tube, then taped over the insertion sight with a cotton ball, instructing each to flex the arm to staunch bloody leakage. Neither said more than 'yes' or 'no' to the phalanx of questions.

Meantime, the ambulance driver was arguing with the gatekeeper to let him out, who refused. Arguing crescendoed into yelling with all three shouting at one another at the same time. When I first witnessed these exchanges, I became concerned they would erupt into violence but they never did. It was common to see this nearly every day amongst the nationals on the job site and around town. Apparently, this was as good as a way to settle disagreements as any in the world. Eventually, everyone would agree on something and quickly deescalate, no lingering hard feelings.

"What are they arguing about, Jabari?" I asked, pointing to the three.

Jabari eyeballed the situation, then remarked, "The gatekeeper wants to know if the sprayer disinfected the ambulance. The ambulance driver and sprayer are saying it was done. But the gatekeeper didn't see it so he wants them to do it over while he watches. The sprayer doesn't want to do it over."

The standoff continued for another two minutes until, finally, the sprayer had enough and, adjusting his nozzle to stream, sprayed at the feet of the gatekeeper who jumped back, stunned, then resumed yelling and shaking his fist. The sprayer and the driver laughed, clearly enjoying their alliance, but this was a mistake. The gatekeeper walked through the gate, pulled the door shut behind him and locked in the ambulance. The driver went silent, then walked to the gate, pushing his face up against the crack and began pleading.

"What's the driver saying?" I asked Jabari.

"He's sorry, so very sorry, and if he opens the gate he will make the sprayer spray the ambulance down again and the gatekeeper can watch," Jabari related.

The driver stepped back and the gate started to open. By the time it was fully opened, the sprayer, who was in back with his hands on the rear door latch, watching from around the rear bumper of the ambulance, slammed the doors shut as the driver hopped into the driver 's seat. With the gatekeeper's back to the ambulance as he swung the gate fully open, the driver stepped on the gas and revved through, getting onto the blacktop free and clear with the gatekeeper yelling hard. The driver leaned out, his toothless laugh in full roar, giving the finger to the gatekeeper as he sped away, who likewise flipped it back to the driver. The gatekeeper turned on his heels, stared down the sprayer and took an aggressive step forward. The sprayer retreated behind the line considered hot zone in the admissions' area, laughing and swinging his spray wand, all the while anonymous in his PPE, taunting the gatekeeper. The gatekeeper had enough, took his lumps and retreated outside the gate doors.

Jabari found all of this hilarious, heaving with laughter. Even the two new patients smiled, amused by the entire spectacle.

Jabari took the opportunity to introduce himself to the two men and explain his role. I assumed I was part of the whole plan but when I started to enter, Gwyn called out to stop me, correcting me, saying, "Rick, don't go with Jabari. He can take care of showing them their beds. I need you to go get...." Gwyn paused, reading the note in her hand, "...Mariatu Conteh, 32 year old female in Confirmed 4. She's a survivor." She handed me the vanilla nametag, a lafa and bar of soap. "You know what to do?"

"Sort of, I think," I guessed. "Bring her out to the shower, get her to clean up, take her to the gate. Someone will be waiting with fresh clothes, right?"

Gwyn congratulated me and sent me on my way. Jabari, with his own two patients, was stopped in the middle of the courtyard by two other anonymous white suits, both with Spanish names on the aprons. Josephine made sure I was wrapped tight. Off I went.

As I walked towards Jabari, I was able to decipher the names on the aprons: Jorge and Alfredo. Jabari was going back and forth with the two fellows when he stopped me, asking, "Rick, you speak any Spanish at all?"

"Nada," I said. "What do they want?"

Jabari, laughing, replied, "I have no idea."

Turning to the two, I tried to unravel the knot, giving it my best shot, asking, "Habla ingles?"

The one marked Jorge spoke, "Little. Si."

"You want to help?" I asked, hoping to solve the riddle of their intentions.

"Help?" Jorge repeated, not sure, then rising up to indicate he understood, going on, "Si, si. Yes, help him," pointing at Jabari and his two patients.

Jabari stuttered, then formed his words, looking at me, "All I'm doing is taking these patients inside. They understand that?"

"I have no idea, Jabari," I remarked, shrugging.

Jabari settled the issue, saying, "Tell you what: you take Jorge and I'll take Alfredo. They're here just to see what's happening today. Maybe it would do some good just to follow. Sound alright?"

I was more than willing to handle my discharge alone, especially since this was my first from Confirmed. I hoped for the opportunity to speak with the patient alone, to explain what she could expect during the process. Trying to explain it to Jorge would be an extra challenge that I wasn't anticipating, but was there really anything to explain that he simply couldn't watch? The answer was that he would be merely shadowing me, observing and figuring it out on his own.

I pointed at Jorge then back to myself, "You. Me." Then I pointed at Alfredo and Jabari. "Alfredo. Jabari." Everyone understood and we split up, Alfredo going with Jabari and Jorge with me.

I put my hand under my name on my apron, getting Jorge's attention, pronouncing my name, "Rick." He nodded his understanding. I continued, showing him the patient's vanilla nametag, emphasizing the letters 'DC' written in bold green, saying, "Discharge. We have to discharge this patient." I also pointed out the latest green markered lab result, the minus sign for negative on Mariatu Conteh's PCR result. "She's….she's…." I stuttered, searching my head for the Spanish, coming up with, "She's bien. Casa. Home. She can go to her casa."

Jorge patiently watched and listened, repeating back to me, "Si. She go home."

"Yes," I enthusiastically confirmed, grateful to know he understood what we were going to do.

We finished the walk across the courtyard and onto the concrete walkway leading to the gate that separated the S and C units. During the walk, I showed Jorge the soap, bucket and clean lafa, hoping he would deduce the patient needed cleaning before her discharge. Through the suit, without a verbal acknowledgement, I couldn't tell if Jorge connected the dots. Now, I wasn't even sure if he was a doctor or nurse.

I petitioned for Jorge's attention at the gate, placing my finger near one of the many nails sticking out, at the ready, to hook a suit and tear it wide open, cautioning him to be watchful, which he acknowledged with an emphatic nod of the head.

Patients were strewn about the front walkway the full length of Confirmed's buildings. Some were listless, wet and foul, oblivious to our arrival. The healthier ones watched us, sitting up with their backs against the walls, watching kids play by the water outlet with some cheap plastic toys brought in for them or listening to the radio. Jorge and I poked our heads into Confirmed 4, trying to spot M. Conteh by age and gender. About a third of the beds had patients in them. Down on the end, a woman sat on her bed, a child between her legs as she wove tight braids and some colored string into a young girl's hair. I walked past the patients, doing my best to lock out their pleas for everything from dry clothes and bedding to pain control, admonishing myself that the discharge was the priority.

At the bed, Mariatu looked up at us, pausing to rest her hands on the girl's shoulders, waiting for Jorge and me to state our business.

"Mariatu," doing my best 'this is good news' tone, "you're test results came back." Triumphantly, I presented her with the vanilla tag, saying, "You're negative. You're well enough to go home. Congratulations."

The little girl, staring up at Jorge and me with her wide, soft brown eyes, mouth frozen, grimacing, began a pout that rolled into soft weeping. She then turned between Mariatu's legs to bury her head in her lap. I wondered if this was Mariatu's daughter.

I softly embraced the girl's arm, feeling bone through her meager flesh, and ran my hand down to her wrist, pulling it up near my visor so I could read her wristband, and read it aloud, "Amimata Fafanah. 7 years old." I looked at Mariatu, asking, "Is this your child?"

Mariatu shook her head softly, half whispering, "No. I have helped take care of her since her aunt left."

My heart sank. I was in no state of mind to inquire if 'left' was a euphemism. Either way, Amimata was on the muddy end of the stick.

Looking at Mariatu, I asked, "Does she know anyone else in here?"

"She plays with some of the other children. I am the only mother she has right now." Mariatu related this matter of factly, going on. "She talks of brothers, sisters and an uncle." Then, in lowered voice, leaning into my ear, states, "I do not ask," shaking her head to drive home the point.

Jorge, standing behind me, sidles up into my line of vision, shaking his head and shrugging his shoulders, indicating his confusion about what is happening. I stand up to explain, "La nina….uhm…no madre?"

Jorge understands. "Malo. Bad."

That certainly sums it up, I thought. I tell Mariatu what we need to do to get her outside the fence and home, handing her a bucket with rags and a lafa. She takes the bucket. Amimata comprehends, falling to the concrete, face down, heaving out sobs. The date on her wristband shows she has been in nearly two weeks herself, testing positive 9 days ago and placed in Confirmed. Most likely, the worst was over for her, would soon test negative and be discharged. Meanwhile, Jorge and I are tearing away Amimata's safety net, her sentry in this death trap, the one person who chased away the monsters lurking under beds and in the shadowy corners.

Others are at the door looking in, most being children with two older women, giving me a chance to make a huge request of them all. A grandmotherly type, her wisdom of a half century etched into her face, looks at me through yellowed and bloodshot eyes. She senses what I am about to ask and disappears. The other woman appears brighter, her eyes clearer. I extend her my appeal to watch over the child, that Mariatu is going home. She listens, frowns, and to my relief, consents to help watch over Amimata. The woman approaches the bed, bends down onto the floor on both knees and picks up the child to her feet, sternly telling her to wipe her tears and that she is now with her, that she will watch over until Amimata is well enough to go home. The two then walked out the door, hopefully to the woman's own mattress and space in another building. I remind myself to tell Musa about this child so he can check her family status.

Mariatu steps in between Jorge and me. I lead both out of the building to the shower through the low, brittle brush. All the plant life is dryer and browner by the day. Due to its 1 yard height, we've taken to calling the water faucet the Gnome Shower. Left over soaps and drying rags are scattered around the concrete basin from other patient discharges. I force myself to resist the urge to start collecting refuse and get on with the task at hand. Jorge and I find a spot of shade along a wall, sitting ourselves down on the curb of one of the deep concrete gutters that was put in to funnel away monsoon waters, next to what looks like was a supply room for whatever it was this place used to be.

Soon enough, Mariatu steps around the corner of the wall, wrapped in the green and yellow lafa we gave her. Outside the fence, out on the drive, a Red Cross/Red Crescent truck is backing down to the morgue to collect the day's failures. They will be delivered to the cemetery for final rights and internment, concrete poured over the bodies to prevent grave theft by those who might insist on a traditional burial. Following the truck is Josephine and one other national, carrying clothes and sandals for Mariatu. Mariatu positions herself at the gate, wordlessly looking on as Josephine eyes Mariatu, sizing her for a best-fit blouse of the five or six she brought with her. Mariatu chooses a flower pattern as the most likely best fitting garment.

Josephine opens her latch on the outside and I remove the bolt from my side. The gate swings open. Speaking in Temne, Josephine has Mariatu drop her lafa but not before admonishing Jorge and I to turn ourselves, to yield some privacy. Josephine permits us to turn back. Mariatu is now dressed in another fresh lafa, her new blouse complimented with red and black sandals accenting the glow of her recovered health. By stepping across the threshold and out the gate, Mariatu will have literally left a black chapter of her life behind a wall of tarps, hardly the most constraining material one could come up with, but that is what we had, 5 millimeters of blue nylon keeping a devastating disease at bay from the rest of the world. I close the gate after Mariatu steps through, then Jorge and I watch the three walk down the driveway, out to the front of the admissions building where Mariatu will have a discharge ceremony. If the two of us get through doffing, we may have a chance to participate.

At the front of the doffing line, Jabari is finished up. To pass time until I'm out, he situates himself on a bench near the worker's prayer mosque, leaving us with no wait. Jorge has Alfredo waiting for him and the two banter back and forth in Spanish, mocking me for all I know, or worse yet, as the joke goes in Hollywood, ignoring me completely. Both of us finish out by scrubbing down our hands and arms, with me waving Jorge and Alfredo to follow to see if we can catch the discharge ceremony.

The four of us hurry down the walkway past workers yelling out greetings, carpenters sawing and hammering, and Ali at the hand washing station asking, for the hundredth time, if I'm going to leave him my boots when I go back to the States. J Edgar et al ask if I want a piece of shade for a minute while they recount the soccer scores they picked up off the radio. We pass George, the sprayers' spokesperson on work issues, and he raises his fist in a solidarity salute, something he picked up from a conversation he and I had on American labor history where I showed him that one finger alone is not as strong as five fingers together that make a fist.

Out in front by the Memory Tree, Gwyn, Dorine and Josephine are working with the four survivors discharged from Confirmed, waiting for their taxi ride back to where home may or may not be, depending on the mood of the village, whether it is fearful or accepting of such survivors' return. In front of each survivor is a pile of goods donated by various organizations to ease the material transition back into everyday life. Many of the patients, living a marginal existence prior to their admission, likely had their personal economy destroyed by their confinement.

Josephine explains in Krio, Temne and English that each survivor receives an eighty-pound bag of rice, two blankets, a mattress, two new high thread count lafas, sandals, cooking oil, 8 liters of bottled water, Paracetamol and 200,000 Leones. Josephine goes on to explain that the van taking the survivors back home will load everything up and help them unload once they arrive back to home, helping them to situate. She goes on to tell the survivors, who wordlessly and patiently listen, expressionless, that their respective chiefs have been contacted. Other workers have spoken to the chiefs to verify that the survivors are welcome back home and are no threat to the safety of the rest of the village. Word had reached back to the hospital that this was not always the case, necessitating Musa to use his indigenous knowledge of local customs to ameliorate the fear and ignorance that surrounded previous survivors, some who returned to their homes to find them burned down, taken or simply barred from return.

Gwyn and Dorine hand each of the survivors a ribbon of colored cloth, welcoming them to tie a bow around a branch as previous survivors had done. The small tree was now becoming more and more prismatic and vibrant with each passing day. Mariatu came forward first, ties her ribbon into a neat bow on a lower branch, then steps back to let the other three each take their turn.

In the final rite before departure, Dorine lines the four survivors up and reads off each name, handing them a laminated Certificate of Cure with the official national stamp embossed in bright blue over the signatures of Dr. George, head of the Maforki ETU, and Rebecca, the nurse matron.

At the conclusion of the ceremony, our small crowd of caretakers and patients let out a cheer, congratulating each survivor just as friends and family back home would applaud a recent graduate. Camera flashes burst as we take turns posing with the survivors, two who accommodate our ceremony but exhibit a tautness revealing their general anxiety over the entire recent experience they endured. Mariatu manages a small smile as her eyes well up. Looking back inside over the fence, gazing for several moments, she then wraps her arms around the other young women who came out with her. The two men were in their teens. If any hint of boyhood came in with them, they were now absolved of their youth and immaturity, men going forward who understood that fate, luck and innocence were more random than predictable and achievable. The driver loads the new belongings, ties the mattresses down to the roof and ushers each one through the waiting door. The van drives off with lives to be concluded somewhere not here.

Off to the side, two other discharges watched the entire ceremony, sitting quietly on the bench. I ask Gwyn, "Why aren't they going with?"

Gwyn pulls me close, whispering, "They're discharges from Suspect that tested negative. They either have to have family pick them up or we give them a little money for motorcycle taxi."

"Motorcycle taxi? How are they going to carry all their stuff, a bag of rice and a mattress on a motorcycle?" I ask, not quiet grasping.

Lowering her voice even more, Gwyn explains, "Suspect cases that test negative get nothing. It was decided that it was not affordable to award discharge gifts to them."

The two middle aged 'survivors', a man and a woman I did not recall treating, continued their wait on the bench under the shade of trees, likely wondering who was going to take them home. After watching the entire discharge ceremony, the substantial compensations for the four confirmed Ebola survivors, I couldn't help but feel terrible, more so because there was no way I could fix it. Their ordeal inside, the dread of awaiting their test results for two days, unwillingly engrossed into the suffering of Ebola infected patients next to them awaiting the same test results that would send them over to the Confirmed buildings. As bad, if not worse, they were in dangerously close proximity to the active infected, their best chance to remain uninfected was to stay put, away from what any of the other patients' touched or fouled. It had to be like walking on blasting caps.

Jabari wandered off inside with Josephine and Gwyn. Alfredo took off down the path to the Cuban station. Jorge finished taking pictures and put his camera back into his knapsack, then pointed at the two remaining patients waiting for their rides, asking, "Superviviente, eh?" After some back and forth between us trying to make sense of one another, it finally dawned on me Jorge was saying 'survivor'. Not wanting to labor over differentiating that someone discharged from Suspect after testing negative was not technically a survivor, I agreed to his understanding, confirming, "Si. Survivor." Jorge ran with this, standing in front of the two Suspect discharges, bursting out, simultaneously flashing two thumbs up and warbling, "Heyyyyyy!". Obviously, the US embargo had not stopped 'Happy Days' from reaching Havana.

I shake my head. "Come on, Fonzy. Time to go home."
■■■

Inconvenienced

Days rolled over into one another with new doctors, nurses and coordinators arriving weekly to try to keep pace with the growing patient loads as teams fanned out into the communities to identify likely Ebola cases that previously were going undetected. The more rural areas were the last to get the news and the last to get the information needed to protect them. Traditional burial rites that involved family and friends washing and touching the body for the final goodbyes continued in spite of educational efforts which, coming from an Apatow, were greeted with suspicion. In neighboring Guinea, several aid workers on educational missions out into the bush villages had their vehicle halted, were dragged out and hacked to death and unceremoniously dumped into a ditch. As far as the attackers were concerned, and many rumors circulated as fact to back them up, it was the Apatow responsible for the dying, coercions from Apatow to change deeply held burial rites, that were part of a scourge they unleashed to control Africans, the same as in the past.

In the larger cities of Port Loko and Freetown, organized contact tracers from the local community were hired to go out house to house to identify the sick as possible Ebola cases and then follow up with who they had contact with over the past three weeks when signs and symptoms of illness first appeared, enabling more effective quarantine precautions. The employment of people from the affected communities afforded the greater advantage of an understanding of the local language and people, many whom the contact tracers knew personally or shared common acquaintances with, something that put people from thousands of miles and completely different worlds at a distinct disadvantage.

Other care workers were being sent out to smaller towns to set up critical care centers, CCC's, and train the national nurses and doctors in safe care technique, with an emphasis on the process of disinfecting with bleach and the proper use of protective personal equipment. Since the epidemic first broke, neighboring Liberia and Guinea, along with Sierra Leone, lost over 300 hundred nurses and doctors. It was a lack of understanding of what they were encountering, preventing them from informed self-protection rather than a lack of having all the proper equipment and disinfectant, followed by simply being overwhelmed with their patient loads, leading to exhausting hours where mistakes in protocol and technique became inevitable.

Maforki became the loci of the Port Loko district fight against Ebola, receiving patients from the far borders where CCC's were not yet up and running or where CCC's were full and had no more room. The influx of arriving patients swelled, with ambulances bringing in as many as 5 patients in one vehicle, usually family. Gwyn now had her own staff of 10 or so to help organize the lab work, history taking, admissions, discharges and the thousand other obstacles and hurdles as unique as each man, woman and child who came or went through the gates.

The previous day had a record 18 admissions to Maforki alone, creating a chain of assessments, treatment plans and new patients to get to know to treat. Protocols on who was placed where, the separating of new dry patients from the new wet patients, created a sense of order along with the turnaround of lab results happening in 24 hours that tested for both malaria and Ebola to further delineate who should get what medicines when.

The supply room was better stocked, making preparations for the first round in easier by being able to check out what we needed from a supply clerk rather than rummaging through stacks of boxes to find antibiotics, antimalarials, analgesics and antiemetics. Nurses and doctors, red biohazard bags full of drugs, syringes and needles, hunkered down in the nurses' station and mixed and loaded Rocephin and Flagyl into syringes, counted IV bags out and matched up IV line. People took turns cutting packets of ORS powder to dump into a 10 gallon plastic trash can, mix, then funnel back into empty 1.5 liter bottles for the patients. Flavorings of cherry, grape and lemon-lime were added to cover up the less than palatable electrolyte solution that was causing more than a few patients to drink much less than needed to stave off the crippling dehydration that came part and parcel with Ebola infection.

Outside the station, a whiteboard hung for team assignments. Beneath the board, wooden stakes had been pounded into the ground to hold boots sole up to dry out between rounds, meaning we weren't digging through a pile of rubber looking for our unique mark to find the right boot for the right foot. Or the right boot for the left foot, too.

Looking at the whiteboard, I found I was on a team with two Cubans, one a doctor and one a nurse and two national nurses along with our building assignment. With admissions coming in at all hours, it wasn't unusual to be called away from over the fence to walk in the new admission and settle them, an extra task for those assigned to Suspect. I looked down to see our building assignment. Suspect.

Knowing the assignment meant running back over to admissions, pulling up a chair jot down on paper the names, sexes and ages of those in our assigned buildings. Next was to check lab results and see if anyone needed to be moved to Confirmed or discharged and to determine what drug protocol they should be started on, such as an anti malaria, antipyretics for fever, IV fluids if unable to take PO or wet and if an IV was in place.

Since there wasn't an adequate system in place to transmit information outside of the fence, one learned to anticipate what drugs and supplies would be needed, prompting us to gather up extra inventory to use for the unexpected or to restock what was short into the medicine boxes Francie and Galleo now managed to get into every building, something in itself that made everyone's job faster instead of hunting and pecking over shelves and tables for the item needed.

Mixing the various medications took about a half hour, measuring out x cc's of saline solution for y medication and outfitting the syringes with needles to avoid having to do so in the contaminated environment of the ETU hot zone saved precious minutes of our allowable time inside to more adequately administer patient cares.

After the morning medication preparations were complete, I walked back to the national nurses' station, knocked on the door and waited for the permission to open, not wanting to walk in on a gaggle of girls trying on each other's clothes. Someone yelled for me to open and come in and on seeing my face, one groaned, "Time already?", flopping back down on her cot and sighing. "OK. Who do you want?"

I always felt like I was imposing upon them, in part because it was never formally established or related to me at least, what the hierarchy was or even if there was a formal one at all. As it stood, what was established and practiced was the aid group I was with fell into place as the lead. Was it due to a power vacuum? Deference to the American reputation of exceptionalism in leading first world responses to third world crisis? My guess was the reason the leadership role fell to us was the poverty of leadership in the nation itself, with far too few trained as managing physicians and nurses spread out beyond thin without adequate funding to establish systems of communication and role ownership. You can't organize and lead what you can't brainstorm and plan.

"Uhm, yeah, I have Isatu and Mary on the schedule for morning round," I related apologetically. "They're here?"

Isatu yelled out from her corner cot, "Oh, Reeck. Of course I go with you. When?"

"Now," I reply.

"Now?", Isatu mocks back. "And Mary? I will find Mary for you. She's hiding from you!" With that, Isatu let out a laugh that the others picked up, speaking in Krio or Temne things that mocked the not present Mary—maybe.

Isatu calmed the riotous laughter, asking in a more serious tone, "Who else is with us today?"

"Two Cubans."

Isatu rolled her eyes, then with exaggerated body language, she rolled again her eyes and slumped her shoulders, groaning, then looked at me, saying, "You know they cannot speak English. You cannot speak Spanish and I cannot speak Spanish and they cannot speak Krio or Temne." Then pausing for effect, blurted out, "We are sooo screwed." With this, the other nurses in the station started screeching and laughing again, taking more than delight in the complication Isatu, Mary, the Cubans and I faced. I could only smile in deference to their observation, shrugging agreement over a situation which was not really in my control or anyone else's. No one wanted to confront the issue of language barriers because that was attached to national and cultural identity and it might seem xenophobic or close-minded to discuss such an issue. While it might have been viewed as politically correct and a noble promotion of the ideal of diverse groups as one team to have us all work together, which it was, it turned a blind eye to the communications issue. On paper it was wonderful but on paper under the column 'possible drawbacks', some bureaucrat penciled in 'none'. It is that man who should be condemned to a lifetime of day after day of customer service calls where the service representative is a monolingual speaker of church Latin.

I left the national nurses' station, letting Isatu round up Mary, and headed next door to the Cuban station to track down the two Cubans on my list, yet again two new faces I needed to meet. Inside some were already dressing for their morning round. Interrupting hesitantly, I called out the names Carlos and Alonzo. No response. Just looks. I repeated myself, dropping the two names out into the room. More stares. Finally, someone mostly geared up came forward, taking my scribbled notes from my hand, deciphering the names, pointed towards the donning station, saying, "Carlos, Alonzo," pointing several more times to emphasize where I should look. I thanked him and walked over to the donning tent, encountering the usual morning rush of tens of bodies donning at once to go in, plastic bags and sticker strips littering the floor as is if someone threw an accidental ticker-tape parade.

I shouted over the voices of the melee inside, "Alonzo? Carlos?" Everyone stopped for a second to look then resumed donning. Not getting a response, I then looked for names on the aprons and hit the jackpot with Alonzo and Carlos quietly waiting in the corner for....me? Laying eyes on one another, I introduced myself, "Mes nombres es Ricardo," then showed them the morning team list. Both nodded vigorously. "OK," I thought, and then continued, "Habla Englais?"

Carlos spoke up, holding his thumb and forefinger, "Little."

There was a one in four chance with 16 Cubans on morning shift, where four spoke passable English, that I would have one English speaker on the assigned team, slightly less than a coin's flip of a chance. I need a two-headed coin.

I showed them the list of patients and related, as best I could, that I would soon be with them. Confident they understood this, I left to get my boots and put an eye out for Mary and Isatu to see if they were on their way, spotting the pair sitting on the walkway putting on their boots. Neither seemed in a particular hurry. Hoping to light a bit of a fire, I told them the Cubans were already dressed and waiting. Both shook their heads, as if wondering what the Cubans' big hurry, or mine, was.

Inside the donning station, the two nationals and I donned as quickly as possible to mitigate Carlos and Alonzo's wait. Zipped and visored, I looked around for the pair of Cubans, not able to see them anywhere.

"Did you see where a Carlos or an Alonzo went?" I asked the man scribbling names on our suits.

"In. They went in with your list," he flatly stated. "Better hurry or they will finish without you." Then he laughed, adding, "They are cheetahs and you are a turtle."

Fine. Mary and Isatu finished donning and off we headed down the walk, arms loaded with waters, medications, rags and no notes on our patients. Inside Suspect 1, a dry ward, Alonzo and Carlos were checking bedside charts and taking temperatures. I saw my notes in Alonzo's hand and lifted his hand up so I could read them, checking to see who had lab results back and could be discharged home or moved to Confirmed. Then I checked to see if we needed to start an antimalaria treatment on any. Two patients were malaria positive and Ebola negative, meaning we would start their antimalaria meds and then ready them for the discharge home, with someone from the admissions team to take them out. I asked Mary to go to the fence to alert the discharge nurse that we would have two ready to go by the time they donned and made it in.

Our next patient was Ebola and malaria positive, meaning we needed to start IV fluids, give a shot of prophylactic Rocephin and start the malaria treatment. He was taking PO on his own but not in any amount adequate for what he was about to go through when the diarrhea and vomiting started. Holding up a bag of IV fluid to help explain what was needed to Carlos, a doctor, and the loaded syringe of Rocephin, and that we then needed to walk the fellow over to Confirmed, Carlos objected in Spanish, shaking his head and saying 'no'. Was he saying no to the Rocephin or no to the IV fluids or no to the antimalaria? I began probing.

I held up the IV bag and Carlos waved his hands and said 'no'. In very hard to understand English and a show and tell display, Carlos grabbed the man's water bottle, putting his finger on the water level to show the man was drinking water on his own, therefore he needed no IV fluids. I then held up the Rocephin syringe and Carlos shook his head 'no', explaining there were no signs of infection. I disagreed. The patient had a fever of 38.9 C, about 102F, evidence of infection. Agreed, it was very likely the Ebola and malaria infections as cause for the fever, but with his body under assault, opportunistic infections normally controlled day to day by a healthy immune system with the patient none the wiser, now had a chance to bloom and further complicate the man's fight to survive, thus the prophylactic antibiotics. I put the loaded syringe back in the bag. Next, I held up the three-day course of antimalaria pills. Here Carlos agreed and he ordered his nurse, Alonzo, to administer the first pills along with 1000 milligrams of Paracetamol for the fever.

This entire episode took a good 10 minutes as Carlos and I attempted to explain our points of view to one another. With Carlos being a physician and me a nurse, a nurse who counted on and trusted the judgment of physicians as a matter of routine back in the States, this made it more difficult for me to push back against his opinion. In my own mind, a report of a patient being able to take PO held very little value since, technically, nearly all the patients could put a water bottle to their own lips and take sips. The problem, the painfully obvious problem, was it was never nearly enough to negate the fluid loss from the diarrhea and vomiting, throwing electrolytes vital to heart and nervous system wildly out of whack, so much that patients became confused and likely succumbed to cardiac arrest when their sodium and potassium crashed. We needed to have IV's in every single patient that walked through these doors and needed to be ready to hang multiple bags a day the moment we observed an inability to keep up their fluid intake on their own.

In the end, I deferred to Carlos the physician. No antibiotics and no IV fluids. I would pass on to the afternoon caretakers my report and likely they would do what I failed to do. For the past several days, it was common to have this type of situation and disagreement over the course of treatment that should be administered. All of this compounded the complexity of delivering fast, best practices care, slowing down what we could do in our allotted time in the hot zone. Eventually, I took advantage of the strict time limit the Cubans were ordered to adhere to and would track back when plausible and follow the advice of the physicians in our group, that being the generous use of prophylactic antibiotics and liberal fluids administration via IV. It was saving lives and for me the proof was the ever increasing number of live discharges vs the in the bag kind.

During this time, Isatu was speaking to the patient in Krio, attempting to explain what we were trying to do and what was going to happen, his transfer to Confirmed and what that meant. The look on the man's face became more and more fractured and depressed. Judging by his looks, Isatu may as well have unrolled a warrant that announced he was about to be hanged.

Mary walked through the metal door to our building, returning from the fence at admissions, telling us the admissions team was busy with others and they wanted to know if we could walk in a new admit to Suspect. I looked at our team's to-do list as if somehow a reason might announce itself with fireworks as to why we couldn't take an admission.

"Isatu," I asked, cranking up my pleading to a grovel, "could you please take this fellow over to Confirmed?" pointing at him and then the patient's name and test results on the list.

My tone revealed my position as weak and Isatu pounced, putting on a bit of a show, "OK, Reeck. But you owe me a Coca-Cola, hmm?"

I agreed. I don't know why; she was able to cut her round short by escorting our new confirmed patient to his new space. He was a walkie-talkie, able to ambulate under his own power, eliminating the jalopy wheelchair that never resided in the same spot, making it a scavenger hunt to find. Isatu helped pack the man's belongings into a dry bucket, led him out the door across the courtyard from bad to worse. Sometimes, I had an overwhelming urge to bring in olive oil and holy water to place on the patient's foreheads and sign the cross, sans Latin. There were issues enough with my own lack of foreign language knowledge without me mutilating a 2,000-year-old religious sacrament.

Meanwhile, Mary waves Alonzo to go with her and they disappear. Carlos and I continue with the remaining patients, using the bedside charts to guide us on what to do next. Fortunately, whether out of deference to me or, like me, he was too tired to struggle with an argument over what should or shouldn't be done. Due to our inability to speak clearly with one another, Carlos went along, even taking the lead to hang fluids and administer pills followed by some water and making sure relevant information was charted so the next team could reference what we'd done on this round. Then our rhythm was interrupted.

"Carlos. Ricardo," Alonzo waves from the door, signaling us to follow. We walk outside with Alonzo leading and get to the admissions fence gate with a small crowd waiting on the other side, engaged in chatter and pointing to an ambulance with its rear doors open. From our vantage point, I, Mary, Carlos and Alonzo see a middle aged man sitting on the ambulance bench, well dressed in fine leather shoes and suit, clutching a travel pack. About 35 years old or so, he tries to project an air of calm, even nonchalance but his constant shifting of the pack in his lap, held close to his torso, gives away his concern. More startling for all of us, the gentleman is not the stereotypical black African patient but looks Middle Eastern. Gwyn, looking perplexed, cuts through the crowd, waving for our attention.

"Rick," Gwyn starts, her hand on her forehead, fingers rubbing her temples, "this gentleman was sent to us from Lungi airport. They are saying he has Ebola symptoms and needed to come here."

"So he's been screened, had blood drawn?" I say guessing.

"No, nothing is done yet," she relates, glancing back into the ambulance. "He was on his way back to Pakistan when he was pulled out of the line at the airport. They noticed he had red eyes."

"Red eyes? He must have a temperature, too, right?", I ask, starting to feel as perplexed as Gwyn. "I suppose we do the usual assessment and go from there."

Two national nurses in full gear had already managed to get the man out of the ambulance and to sit in a waiting chair under the shade of the admissions' area tarp. One of them starts to ask the routine assessment questions in English but his comprehension is limited. After several tries of questions and acting out various symptoms, the fellow catches on, appearing to give adequate and reliable answers of yes or no. In fact, I heard only one yes and that was to the headache question. He denied contact with any known Ebola patients or that he even was in Ebola infected areas, denied diarrhea, vomiting, fatigue, weakness, nausea, generalized pain or feeling feverish. One of the nurses placed the scanning thermometer to his head and it came back as 100.0, possibly likely due in part to the warm ride in the back of a windowless ambulance for the last 2 or 3 hours.

Carlos watched intently as did Alonzo and Mary, waiting for Gwyn to make her announcement. I ask one of the assessing national nurses to hold up the clipboard at the fence so we can all read it, with Mary, Carlos, Alonzo and I taking our turns going over the information, noting the man's name as Shahid Gola, 34, from Hyderabad, Pakistan. The only two items remotely positive for possible Ebola symptoms are the headache and red eyes, which could be a hundred things, the least of not which could be fatigue and stress from his travel schedule which, judging by his attire, was likely a business trip crammed in between other business trips. The shoes were slip- ons and no metal belt buckle and the pack was pretty typical of what was considered recommended for quicker screening of carry-on bags, all to make zooming through security lines more efficient.

Carlos bumps me with his elbow, getting my attention, and shakes his head 'no'. I understood immediately what he meant, that the fellow had no business being sent here and certainly had no business being admitted.

Gwyn, yards away and pacing the admissions perimeter, puts her phone down and yells for Jabari and Musa to come out, then she puts the phone back to her ear, continuing the call. Jabari and Musa hop out of the building and Gwyn ends her call, relating the story of the patient who was now Curious Object 1 in the compound, a man who never should have been sent on a 2-3 hour ride in an Ebola ambulance and delivered into the hot zone admissions area.

As Gwyn, Musa and Jabari huddle, they appear to reach the same conclusion that Carlos had reached, shaking their heads 'no'. All three walk to the fence to speak with my team on the other side. Gwyn starts by saying, "He shouldn't have landed here but now we have him."

"There's a lot of questions how this happened but our job is to get him out of here and home," Musa states, looking at Shahid who is looking back, knowing he is the subject.

Jabari, arms crossed, devoid of his perpetual smile, looks at the ground, states the predicament well, saying, "He never should have made it this far or at the least been kept in Freetown. Why he was sent here is a mystery. But here he is, his risk increased by riding in the back of an Ebola ambulance and dropped off in the admitting hot zone."

"We can't turn the ambulance around. They can't do that because he's got other scheduled pickups today taking him further out," Musa explains, having spoken with the driver briefly prior to our huddle.

Now we just all start looking at one another and eventually Gwyn feels our collective agreement that Shahid should not be here and that we need to get him out toute suite. It's her call. Do we admit him into a Suspect building and then work on his discharge? Treat him like any other patient, admit him, pull his blood and wait for results that, likely negative, would be the golden stamp of approval that he was OK and safe to travel?

Gwyn, not wanting to rush a decision that was going to have complications and implications no matter how it was handled, looked at each of us, asking what we'd do.

Everyone agreed Shahid did not belong here, that he did not meet the assessment criteria for admission. However, he was ours and now had some incidental and brief contact in a high risk Ebola area, meaning we couldn't just send him out the door to find his own way back to the airport and get another plane out. Carlos grasped the content of the discussion, objecting to Shahid going any further but also seemed to understand that kicking the man out the front gate wasn't a viable option either. Finally, Gwyn, took ownership.

"Rick, can you clean up a space in Suspect for him and keep him away from the rest of the patients?" Gwyn asked.

Mary stepped forward to field the question for me, replying, "There are two private rooms in Suspect 1 that no one has been in. Send a sprayer in to re spray and make sure it is disinfected."

"And have someone in clean PPE who hasn't been inside today," Musa interjected, continuing, "you guys have been hands on already. Someone clean can walk him in."

Jabari nodded his agreement, paraphrasing Musa and Mary, "Yes, get him into a clean room away from everybody and make certain whoever walks him in isn't anyone who's been in yet today," pointing to us on the other side of the fence. "We keep him as clean as we can."

Carlos then grabbed our attention, extending his left arm and using his right hand to slap the traditional blood draw site for testing, emphasizing we needed to get his lab results.

Gwyn looked at Carlos, speaking louder than normal, "Yes, Carlos, I'll get his labs drawn right away and see if we can get a stat on it, see if we can get it back by this evening." Then turning to the whole group, Gwyn gave us her plan, including what we had agreed on, and the phone calls she'd be making to fix the mess Shadid was in now.

Mary had already left to collar a sprayer to prep the room and Jabari decided he would be the one to don PPE and walk Shahid into the ETU. Carlos, Alonzo and I were ready to return when Carlos once again turned my attention with an elbow bump, and pointed at Shahid.

"No," I said, misunderstanding, "we won't be walking him in. Someone else will do that."

Carlos shook his head in a way that I misunderstood his intent, and digging deep for English, spoke, "Shahid. Must know."

He was right. Someone needed to do their best to bring Shahid up to speed on the plan. With none of us able to speak Arabic and Shahid's English apparently limited, one of us would have to try to make him understand our intentions. Then one of my better ideas popped into my head.

"Hey, Gwyn," I shouted, as she was on her way back inside, "can someone write down what the plan is and give it to Mr. Gola. Sometimes people are better at reading a foreign language than they are at hearing it. Can we give that a try? This poor fellow needs to know what we're doing."

Gwyn looked back at me, thinking maybe I was a bit daft for not realizing that she'd already thought of it, then smiling, "Ok. We can try that."

"So you're good then," I asked, trying to bow out.

"Yes. Go ahead."

I looked at Shahid in his chair. He was still holding his bag tight and I then realized that most likely he was carrying very important items like his passport, plane ticket, wallet, money, phone, laptop, camera and other essentials and valuables. Technically, it was now in the hot zone and technically, it could not be let out again. It would have to be destroyed and burned. At that thought, I swore at myself, angry about a problem we really had no power to solve. To avoid ruminating on it, I excused myself that several more patients were waiting inside for us to finish. Over 90 minutes had passed and Carlos and Alonzo were violating their Cuban protocol and I wasn't feeling very comfortable in my gear, starting to slobber up in my mask and feeling the familiar squish of sweat soaked socks in my boots. Mary was visibly uncomfortable, sweat rolling down into her eyes, causing her to shake her head to maneuver it away, unable and verboten to use her gloved hands to try to wipe it away.

We all re-entered where we left off and made quick work of the remaining two patients, and headed for the doors when Jabari came through with Shahid. Jabari stopped, looking over at us as we tied up loose ends, asking, "Hey, Rick, who exactly is in charge? I mean, this poor fellow doesn't belong here and Gwyn's out there making a hundred phone calls to get this all straightened out. This is something that should be settled immediately, not in 12 or 24 hours and certainly not with him inside here."

I was caught off guard, thinking I was the only one who was quietly wondering the same thing. Satisfied with allowing myself to follow the advice and lead of the physicians and fellow nurses, a group I trusted, in fact the only group I trusted, as I was able to witness and hear their various arguments for what we should or should not do. It's hard to hold close to your bosom the ideas of those you are not able to have regular and conversant contact with, a phenomena studied to death in business schools and politics where it has been found that the further from the decision making processes a worker or citizen is, the more likely they are to distrust directives and policies from the top. Dr. George was titled head of our hospital and thus under the control of the Ministry of Health. But he was rarely seen on site since he had other duties such as overseeing the government hospital in Port Loko and clinics in surrounding communities. For guys like me, it was the Major, Galleo, Peterson, Kelli, Brett and Francie who became defacto leaders, experts by dint of either being physicians or having been at Maforki the longest.

So all I could do was mumble back at Jabari, "Sure in the hell ain't me."

Jabari laughed, but it was a dead serious laugh laced with sarcasm. "Yeah, well," changing the subject back to Shahid in the present, "this room right here is going to be his."

The room had a door, a brand new mattress, and a real sheet was in the admission bucket along with two lafas and a heavy blanket, water, a candy bar someone must have donated and minor drugs such as Paracetamol. The patient, resigned to it all, followed Jabari's direction and allowed Jabari to arrange his bed and set things up in an arranged order on a nearby table. Outside Shahid's window, he could look out onto the admissions area and see what was happening. Jabari emphasized that Shahid should stay in his room to avoid risking more exposure than he already experienced. I could see Shahid acknowledging these instructions with a nod of his head, meaning he grasped at the least the basics of what was happening to him.

As for the rest of our group, language barriers definitely slowed us down as a team. I felt responsible for their safety, to point out the hazards like nails, pieces of scrap tin, slivers of wood and other harmful protuberances waiting to ambush any one of us should we let down our guar. The others went ahead but I remained behind to check on how our patient we sent from Suspect to Confirmed was doing.

The patient was settled on his bed in C-4, back to the door, lying down. He had not touched his water since our first contact earlier. I grabbed his water, undid the lid, and held it near his cracked lips, trying out my best Krio, "Wata." He turned his head up, letting me put the bottle to his mouth, taking some in as I tipped out the water but stopped, refusing to take more. This wasn't good. And I wasn't going to wait until he became more ill to start an IV, something we should have done over in Suspect before we sent him.

At the building's medicine box, I rummaged through what was once a neatly arranged box where everything was easy to find but was now a mixed up pixy-stix pile of med packets, cotton, tapes, needles and syringes. After a few minutes, I found a 20-gauge needle, IV line and a bag of IV fluid lying on the floor, intact in its wrap.

At the bed, I showed the patient my supplies then pointed at the needle, pointing to the nice large vein on his left arm and then pointed out the several other nearby patients with running IV's so he'd understand what I was going to do. He nodded his assent and rolled on to his back, giving me his left arm. I went back to the door and found the bleach bucket, pushed the button and....nothing. I tipped the bucket towards me, getting the remnants to the faucet, dousing each hand then vigorously scrubbing for a good minute. Back at the bed, I set up the bag and line, ran the fluid to fill the line and clamped it off to be at the ready for the IV start.

Unpacking the needle, which was not a safety needle like one would find back in the States, one that was designed to retract the metal needle at the push of a button into a safety sheath to minimize the risk of an unwanted stick that could transmit a patient's possibly diseased blood to the clinician. No, this needle was raw and fixed, meaning once the plastic catheter was placed in the patient, the metal needle used to help poke into the vein would be exposed and with no safety guards once withdrawn. It was an unacceptable item, this type of IV needle, but it was all we had. It would be easy to say our complaints about this fell on deaf ears but our superiors were often clinicians themselves, thus knowing better and full well the increased risk of an unwanted stab.

With both of us ready, I counseled the patient, "You'll feel a sting, like a small bee maybe. Please, try not to move."

"OK," he agreed, reflexively creating a fist for me as I wrapped the blue tourniquet above his elbow to pop the vein on his forearm. A nice, easy fat one. As I placed the needle at a 20 degree or so angle then touched the vein, he reacted strongly, startling me enough that the needle fell from my fingers. Instinctively, I reached to keep it from falling off the bed to the floor. Terrible move. I managed to stop the needle from bouncing away and at first felt what I thought was a stick, causing me to yell out, "Goddamn it!" I slowly lifted my palm the needle was under, seeing the needle end was out of the boundary of my hand and that the stick I was feeling was the hard plastic lip of the female end of the IV catheter. "Lucky bastard," I thought, "you stupid, lucky bastard."

I regrasped the needle and eased the patient back to ready, though he was a bit sheepish over what had happened but now was more determined not to let his trepidation govern his reactions. With a slow move, I dimpled the skin over the vein, pinning it to keep it from rolling away and pushed the sharp end through the vein wall, getting the red flash. Evenly and slowly, I moved the needle further up the barrel of the vein the full length until the hub of the IV was placed flush and the catheter was fully in. In the meantime, the young man grimaced but was resolute not to flinch or move his arm, sucking it up with no sound crossing his blue lips. I pulled the needle back and tossed it into the biohazard box, took my finger pressure finger off the vein above the IV and saw good blood flow, attached the IV line, opened it and watched the drip rate in the drip canister. It was a fast, even drip so I set the clamp to allow the bag to take about two hours to run out. I applied one more piece of tape, a task that meant peeling it off my gloves carefully so as not to rip them, another hazard of IV placement inside the ETU.

Standing up and gathering the trash, I announce to the patient, "We got it. You're good to go. Try to keep drinking." I throw away the garbage and turn back to grab his chart to document the first bag of fluid. He is watching the fluid run down the line and into his arm but then looks up at me, asking, flatly, "Am I going to live?"

In the three weeks I was now at Maforki, not once had I heard that question from a patient. In the states doctors and nurses heard it all the time and usually appropriately so from cancer or other seriously ill patients. It is a question fraught with all sorts of truthful answers that are unpleasant, forcing half-truth answers to soften the edges that end up being worse than an honest one.

I stare back at him, then blurt out. "I think you will," meaning it. "You have your age and otherwise good health going for you. That seems to be the best chance. Two weeks ago those that came in here were already too sick and too far gone to be able to help," lying to him when it was the lack of appropriate treatment due to a lack of supplies and manpower that was partly responsible for the appalling 90% mortality rate. "You got here early in your sickness and that makes a big difference. What I need from you is for you to drink. We're going to run IV fluids as much as we can and give you other medicines to help out. Protect that IV line like your life depends on it because it does."

Taking it all in, he keeps his flat affect, then quietly asks, looking at the bed next to his, "Do I have to stay next to that man?"

In all the haste of trying to start his line and get myself out, I never even noticed his patient neighbor. I walk over to the bed and place my hand on the man's neck, looking for a carotid pulse. Even with two layers of gloves, I can feel the coolness of death through the gloves. Both his eyes were wide open with not even the common death look, the half droop of the eyelids. His eyes were moist and mostly clear. I pull the man's lafa over the full length of his body.

I turn back to my patient, saying, "I'm sorry, so sorry. I'll move you into another bed in the building next door. It will be awhile before they can move him."

I gather his belongings into a dry bucket for him to carry while I handle the IV bag, holding it up as we walk out. With bad going to worse, a large woman stretched prone on the concrete front walkway, her clothes soaked in her own filth, mumbles unintelligibly, her hand grabbing at my boots. The entire length of her body covers the width of the walkway, forcing us to step over her. She grabs again hard enough to stop my forward motion as I cross her, nearly tripping both the moving patient and me. Luckily, the fellow has the presence of mind to use the wall to keep us upright on our feet. Seeing another white blob of PPE down the walk, I yell down the walkway, "Hey, can you come and see what this woman wants. She's not looking good. I'll help you get her back in bed when I get this patient settled."

The blob with no name on the apron, yells back, "Not my patient." It then turns away and takes its place in the doffing line.

More stunned than angry or disappointed by being blown off, I get my patient into his new bed, next to two other young men his age and in about the same condition, hoping they can support each other through their ordeal.

Back outside, I go back to the woman on the walkway. In her blue dress and blue and gold head wrap, she sees me as I kneel down on the walk next to her and grab her shoulders to try and prop her up against the wall into a sitting position. Her weight makes her an anomaly in here, meaning I was usually able to lift a majority of patients, most who were lighter than my own 150 lbs. Not her. I pushed again on her shoulders, inching her up against the wall. Now she was quiet. Her head flopped to one side, her eyes in a fixed stare. Sweating harder and challenged for breath, I mutter the plain seen, "Fuck, man. She's dead."

I get off my knees and sit on the concrete, next to my new found corpse, who flops back against my shoulder like she's a prom date, her head on my shoulder. I look down at the doffing line going out. Most everyone is finished. It's time to go and inform the corpse team that there are two bodies for them to take care of. When I stand up and look across the fence back into Suspect over the courtyard, I see Shahid through a window looking straight back at me, then wonder if he watched me wrestle with this body, further creating more unneeded anxiety in his already stress filled situation. For all he knew, he was looking at what his future could be in two weeks, a risk we increased the moment we opened the front gate to allow the ambulance carrying him inside to the dirty admissions area.

After I lifted myself off the ground, the body leaning on me slid back down. I grabbed a drying lafa out on the laundry stones. This does the job to cover her up, allowing me to head to the doffing station. The kids are playing on dirty mattresses that need to be disinfected, or had been, and are laid out in the sun to dry. The scene of the kids reminds me of the 'Lord of the Flies', leaving me to wonder if I should judge them as being blissfully naïve or morally indifferent to the suffering they were diagnosed as being part of. Or it could be denial, the ubiquitous mental shield for all things bad. My guess was that these children went through the worst of it and were waiting to get back a negative result to be discharged.

As I stood spread into a cross during the spray down, the coolness of the bleach water pealed the heat off of me, providing instant relief and that I was only a short 10 minutes away from being out of this plastic bag and under a fan drinking an icy water. Time for lunch.

■■■

Shovels, Dust and Photographs

The ETU was busier by the day as more and more patients arrived from all directions, giving us   a sense that things were not under control as much as we'd like to imagine. However, our view was skewed by the fact that Maforki ETU was made into the loci of patient Ebola treatment, meaning we took all overflow from the outside areas and CCC's. A visit to the admissions building revealed just how fast things were moving as Gwyn and her crew were juggling phones to make the connections to get Object A to fit into Hole B.

Morning report was a flurry of activity and new information and patients having to move from Suspect to Confirmed or discharged out for testing negative. The triaging of the patients into wet and dry along with 24 hour lab results was a vast improvement in ETU logistics. The Major and Kelli now had several new recent arrival nurses to help them cover the growing pediatric responsibilities, a good overlap since the Frontier 4 were set to rotate out before Christmas back to the states, their assignment fulfilled.

With morning report notes in hand, I contemplated the day's plan of action to get patients moved between buildings, treated and discharged. This morning J Edgar was in a black sweater to fend off the chill lingering from overnight. Motorcycle travelers on the main road were in winter coats, some of them sporting NFL logos with a few displaying Chicago Bears or Green Bay Packer colors like you'd see in the northern states in the thick of winter. I asked J Edgar if he'd ever seen snow and he replied that cool nights like the last were bad enough so why on earth would he want it to be so cold that rain froze. I told him that it isn't Christmas season without a fresh new snow making the world quiet under a soft winter blanket, a white so pure that all the nicks and scars of nature are removed, leaving the forests and fields to slumber and dream of spring buds and flowers.

"Mr. Reeck," J Edgar replied, "Christmas is best under a palm tree. No one freezes to death under a palm tree or needs to huddle around a fire. I've seen your Christmas pictures. Everyone looks cold," he concludes, shaking his head at such silliness. And he's sort of right, I think, no one has ever had heart attack shoveling sunshine.

Ali, his usual good natured self, stops everyone coming in and records their temperature, making certain that their shoe soles are sprayed and hands washed. While I'm washing my hands, he taps my Wal-Mart work boots with his rubber booted foot, asking, "I get those when you leave, correct?"

"Only you, Ali. No one else. But I did get an offer of 300,000 Leones for them," I say, trying to get a rise out of him.

He looks back at me, dangling his thermometer in his hand, worried, then replying with disappointment in his voice, saying, "I cannot pay that."

Seeing that I took this too far, I reassure Ali, saying, "I'm joking, Ali. If anyone offered me 300,000 for these boots I'd only take it to buy a new pair for you and give you the left over Leones stuffed inside. Don't worry; your name is on them."

Inspecting my boots, then looking up at me, Ali replies, "I don't see my name anywhere. It is inside the boot?"

Laughing at his literalness, I tell him it's a figure of speech. He isn't impressed.

"Can you put my name on them now? So no one else takes them?"

His determination to have my boots is unsettling but only for a moment until I remind myself that the chances are remote of finding boots like I'm wearing for sale in Sierra Leone. He needs to be reassured I'm good for this deal. "You have a magic marker in your drawer there." I plop my foot up on his recording table next to our names and temps for the day. "Write your name on the cuff," I instruct.

Ali grabs a black marker out of his drawer and stoops over for a good view, spelling out A-L-I on both boots. His expression is one of a satisfied relief. The boots are as good as his when I leave.

The whiteboard on the nurses' station is down on the ground, moved to accommodate the expansion of the station to make room for the extra bodies joining us and to give us room to organize the place in the future. As it stands this morning, the nurses' station is a state of utter chaos with boxes of PPE, blankets, office supplies, our respective school packs, notebooks, water bottles empty and full, syringe barrels, biohazard boxes, various medications, old notes and sand littering the plastic checkerboard floor covering, gouged and torn from weeks of use. A gecko eyeballs me from the window frame. I name him and give him the sign of the cross, telling him to put no stock in my blessing as I'm not St. Francis and can't protect him from the Minister birds calling the ETU home base. He had no expectations of me having useful powers, shrugs and scampers off do something more entertaining.

Banging and sawing is going on over head as the addition's frame is finished off by three or four carpenters while below several others are moving sand into level for the future pouring of a concrete ramp and porch, doubling the size of the space. I navigate the nails and rough pieces of lumber being used for forms, structure and bracing.

The whiteboard has the day's assignments but my name is absent. Maybe they have another job for me today. Inside, I track down Dennis and he tells me that it was an oversight. We both review who is doing what where and it appears to be well covered, so I offer a solution, offering, "Let me and a national nurse go in and take over everyone else's discharges. It frees them up to focus on patient care and saves everyone a ton of running back and forth." I had an ulterior motive, that being I would be avoiding the stress of a large team with language issues. Handling the discharges with a national nurse would be straight forward and create an easy to use point of contact on the inside for the admissions building staff to work with. Win-win-win.

Dennis squints at the board, "Mmmmm.....yeah. OK. But you have to get a hold of the teams and tell them you're handling their discharges, OK?"

"Gothcha'," I say, pumping thumbs up. I run back to the admissions building and jot down all the discharges Gwyn has assigned on their whiteboard and tell her that for the morning, a national and I will be handling the discharges. Judging by her enthusiasm, life was just simplified for all of us as she rounded up the gate team that would receive the discharges at the gate, telling them about my assignment and that I'd be starting in the next half hour.

With that settled, I ran back to the national nurses' station, waving to the calls of "Reeck!" as I run past J Edgar and the snoozing sprayers benched up against the shade of the blue tarps. On the whiteboard, I see Dorine is assigned to a team of seven, three of them national nurses. I erase her name and rewrite hers and mine as a team.

"Dorine," I say, knocking on their door, "you and me are doing the morning discharges."

She yells for me to come in. Most everyone has gone somewhere else, a couple of nurses playing on their cell phones or video players. "Just you and me?" she asks.

"Yeah. You and I will be doing the discharges. Nothing else. Ready to go now?"

"OK" Dorine replies, unimpressed.

I go through the nurses' station and Dennis is already a step ahead for me, gathering up the discharges everyone else has on their lists and putting them together on a separate list. We compare our lists, satisfied it will work fine.

Then I notice the name: Shahid Gola, the Pakistani from yesterday. But no test result.

"Dennis," I say, pointing out the name, "remember this Pakistani from yesterday? He has no test result. We can't discharge him unless they have a negative PCR, right?"

Dennis focuses on the name, his mental wheels turning. "You're right. We can't let him go."

"But here's part of the problem," I say, trying to bring him up to speed on what he likely already knows, "he was stopped at Lungi Airport for having red eyes. No other signs or symptoms, yet he ended being sent here for God only knows, dropped into the admissions receiving area. We had nowhere else to put him."

Dennis replied, slightly exasperated, "I know that. I'm just wondering why there's not a test result. He doesn't even have a PLK number."

I grab my phone out of my backpack, dialing up Gwyn. "Hey, Gwyn, on Shahid Gola, the Pakistani, there's no test result but he's down for discharge. He doesn't even have a PLK number. Did he get drawn?"

Gwyn explains a convoluted story. I decide that the Major should hear it first hand, handing him my phone. He listens, nodding and mumbling his understanding. He hands the phone back to me, disconnected. "The Dutch refused to assign a PLK, saying he did not meet the admission criteria, that he shouldn't be here in the first place, so there was no reason to draw his blood. Gwyn says the SL embassy and Pakistani embassy are ironing out the details for his transportation back to Pakistan. He's good to go."

I'm thinking this is too easy. Then Dennis looks at me, smiling at my doubt and the opening it gives him to say, "Hey, how hard could it be."

"We're going to find out," I shoot back at him, chuckling.

Dorine is in the doffing tent, half dressed. I hurry to catch up with her then show her the list of names. Six morning discharges. Three from suspect and three from confirmed. Finishing up zipping ourselves in, we take off down the walkway into Suspect with me telling her about Shahid Gola and that we should get him out first. While she gets him ready, I'll communicate across the fence into admissions who we will bring out first so they're ready with fresh clothes at the gate.

Dorine peels off to Suspect to prep Shahid and I go to the fence, telling Josephine we're bringing one man out first. She hands me the discharge bucket of soap, rags and lafa covering and I head over to the shower faucet, watching Dorine bring Shahid across the courtyard. He has his bag and looks none the worst for the misplaced ordeal put upon him. Now the real fun begins, I'm thinking, telling him he can't take his bag out the gate.

Shahid arrives at the faucet, and handing him the bucket, showing him the soap, I then point for him to turn on the water, acting out he needs to strip his clothes and bathe. Shahid hesitates, than shakes his head in the negative, pointing at Dorine.

"I think he wants you gone. He's being a little shy," I tell Dorine.

"Like I really want to see a strange man shower," she sniffs. "I go get the other two ready to come out."

"Good idea," I agree, glad it's smoothed over.

Shahid takes off his clothes, which I reach to pick off the ground and put into a refuse pile, then stop myself, realizing I've touched nothing, and want to keep it that way as long as possible should I have to help dress someone. Shahid runs the water, placing his hand under the running water until he's satisfied that it is tolerable. With no hesitation he squats beneath, getting his whole frame underneath and soaking his jet black shoulder length curly hair and the rest, taking the soap bar and lathering himself, scrubbing with a vigor that suggested a fear of contamination. After the first lathering and rinse, he starts up again, redoing the entire process over just as vigorously. When it looks like he's about to start a third round, I stop him with a wave of my hands and a shake of my head, holding up his drying lafa and offering it to him. Shahid takes the coarse cloth to use as a towel then tries to hand it back to me. I wave him off again and act out he should he wrap himself in it and point to the sandals he should put on to walk to the gate.

At the gate, Josephine and one other national have clothes for Shahid. I see Gwyn trotting down the drive outside the fence, waving. She gets to the gate, catching her breath. "They don't want him to leave just yet."

Not surprised, I ask, "Why not? He's not supposed to even be here."

"They want his blood drawn. The Pakistanis are nervous about him coming back into the country."

I point out what Gwyn already knows, saying, "Draw blood for what? He's symptom free. His eyes aren't even red anymore. No fever. No contact. He hasn't even been in a part of the country with an outbreak. The only people with a lower risk profile live in another country. The longer he stays in here the more likely he is to come in contact with something that could infect him."

Grasping the wire fence between us, Gwyn looks at me, saying, "We know but they're uncomfortable without some medical reassurances."

Crap. "How we going to do this?" I ask.

Gwyn shakes her head, continuing, "We draw and wait for results."

Frustrated, I sigh, "Man, that just doesn't work for me. Or him." In the pause of searching for something to add, I have an idea, continuing, "If they need medical assurance, how about using the Certificate of Health that declares discharges Ebola free. It's signed off by medical staff. He gets one, right?"

"Yes, he gets one," she assures me. Then she rationalizes on Shahid's behalf, saying, "that document is a medical reassurance Number One."

I pick up her rationalization, running with the ball, "No one asked specifically for a blood draw to show negative is my guess. They just want an assurance he's negative."

Gwyn laughs. "Yeah."

I see Dorine at the faucet washing up the next two slated for discharge. Josephine and her colleague shuffle back and forth on their feet, bored, wanting to get on with it all. I ask Josephine to open the gate latch from the outside and as she does this, two white figures appear from around the corner of the building between Shahid, the shower and me. I see Dr. Galleo's name scrawled on one apron and Dr. Castro scrawled on the other.

Straight to the point, Dr. Galleo asks, "Why's he still here?"

"You know about this?" I ask, surmising correctly Galleo's presence has something to do with some sort of hiccup at the national hospital in town and he wasn't needed there, putting him here.

In his own curmudgeonly way, Dr. Galleo mocks me, saying, "If I didn't know about this why would I ask why he's still here," shaking his head at my thick headedness.

Gwyn jumps to my defense and starts explaining the story and the snags. Dr. Galleo listens intently, waiting for the whole story, considering all the factors thoughtfully before forming his conclusions. After Gwyn finishes, Galleo responds, "That national Certificate of Health declaring him Ebola free isn't predicated on a blood draw alone. That only matters when a person fits the admission criteria or has tested positive at least once and is now negative, sign and symptom free. Since he never had the symptoms," his voice rising to emphasize the correctness of his conclusions, "he doesn't need a negative blood draw. What needs to be done now is that since he was in a high risk area, the Pakistanis need to put him under 21 day quarantine when he gets home. He's not sick. He's no danger to anyone on the plane. Give him the certificate."

Castro, listening patiently, backs up Galleo, saying in perfect English I was never lucky enough to get when assigned with the Cubans, "He never belonged here. He is fine and is a danger to no one. Keeping him here longer is a danger to him. Let him go.

Dr. Galleo is direct and firm, ordering, "Open the gate."

Josephine unlatches the gate from her side and lets it swing out towards her.

"Do you have everything to dress him with?" Galleo asks, impatience in his voice.

Josephine, sensing Galleo's prickly nature, responds with her own slight bristling, "Of course. We're not stupid."

Galleo catches how his tone is coming off, and apologizes. "I did not mean to imply anything like that. I know you know what to do."

Galleo motions for Shahid to the gate. I think he's going to try and explain to Shahid the holdup but Galleo places Shahid at the door, steps behind him and asks, "Ready?" giving Shahid a commanding but gently controlled push in the middle of his back on the lafa wrap. "Now tell him to drop the lafa and Rick will pick it up to throw away in here. Everyone see how easy that was. Send the Pakistanis our best wishes."

Shahid, looking startled, quickly grabs at the clothes Josephine is holding out. He races to put on the pants to cover himself then just as quickly pulls over a t shirt. The pants are at least two sizes too large. Shahid sees this and rolls up the cuffs several times to uncover his feet then pulls at the ill fitting t shirt, clearly not happy with its oversize. Gwyn assures him that they'll look for better clothes.

Shahid turns, remembering his bag, pointing at it. Galleo shakes his head empathically, saying, "Sorry. The bag has to stay."

A look of panic comes over his face, fumbling with his tongue, he finally manages, "Passport."

We all look at one another. Galleo yells out, "Sprayer!" From across the courtyard an idle sprayer walks over and asks what we want.

"Rick, go through that bag and see what we can spray and get through the fence to him. Anyone have plastic baggies?" Galleo asks.

Josephine, prepared by previous experience of patient's wanting the SIM cards out of their phones spared, produces a handful of plastic baggies from her pockets.

I unzip the 30 pound travel bag and pull out neatly packed clothes, hygiene items, a laptop, smart phone, Shahid's wallet with ID, a solid handful of cash and passport.

"You're hands clean?" Galleo asks.

"I haven't touched anything until now," I tell him.

"Well, you should have washed down before you ripped into that bag," Galleo replies, instructing me to do so now.

I wash and then he directs me to take the passport and phone and put them into the baggie first. I do this and Galleo then tells me to lay out the plastic covered ID and cash, telling the sprayer to mist them. The sprayer does this and I flip the items to so he can get the other side.

"Put them in the bags, too," Galleo instructs me. "Now seal them. The bleach on the other items will be enough to disinfect the other two in the bag." Galleo looks at Shahid, talking loudly, "One hour," holding his finger up. "In one hour you can take those things out of the bag and use them again," then apologetically continues, saying, "the other things cannot leave the hot zone. I'm sorry."

Shahid indicates he understands and Gwyn, Josephine and her colleague escort Shahid away, down the dusty drive.

Galleo turns to Castro, pointing at me, "Castro, you have to keep on these male nurses."

Castro laughs, agreeing, "Si."

I shake my head, defending myself with a like insult, "Your med students must just adore you."

"If I wanted them to adore me, I'd make them build a shrine to me in the on-call room," Galleo shoots back, asking, "You need any more help?"

I tell him no.

"We didn't come over to help with your discharges." Galleo is serious now. "What we need to know is, did you discharge an 8 year old boy?"

Dorine brings her two discharges from the shower to the gate and I step aside to give the three of them room for their final disrobing and dressing.

Distracted by my own discharges, I answer Galleo. "No. We have no 8 year old boy. No kids at all. Why?"

Galleo and Castro both shake their heads in disbelief. Galleo relates more of the issue to me and Dorine, waving us closer in out of earshot of the discharges Josephine is giving instructions to as they dress to leave. "There is an 8 year old boy by the name of Mariatu Sesay. He was here with his mother but she passed a couple of days ago. Mariatu was getting well, well enough he was outside playing with the other kids yesterday. The lab crew was supposed to draw blood on him to see if he was ready for discharge but couldn't find him. Everyone just assumed he moved from one building to another on his own like they do sometimes."

I have nothing to offer except speculation and say so. "I have yet to discharge any kids at all. Even if he left with any of the other discharges you'd think someone would notice a kid. Were there any families discharged with kids he could have latched on to and are we sure he was here yesterday?"

Castro interjects, fleshing out our problem. "His bed chart shows that he was seen yesterday morning and yesterday afternoon."

Normally with discharges, you immediately take their bedside chart notes and put them away under the med cabinet with a note written across the face 'Discharged' to avoid chasing around a phantom patient who is gone either way. Per Castro, that's not the case.

Galleo offers an answer to my questions, speculating himself, saying, "Our record keeping is challenging but it's pretty clear he was here yesterday if someone recorded a temp for him. No families have been discharged en masse as of yet I know of or anyone else knows of. If you have time, can you walk around the grounds and take a look to see if he's hiding somewhere. We're looking as we do rounds and we'll look some more."

"Yeah, of course I'll look." Then I add, "Do Gwyn and Musa know about this at all? Maybe the kid ended up shipped off to one of the orphanages. They know all the drivers who take these patients back to their villages. They'd have to remember an 8 year old kid you'd think."

"Musa and Gwyn already are making phone calls. We were just at the fence asking them what they knew," Galleo confirms, continuing, "Everyone's looking. We gotta' go and finish up."

With that, Galleo and Castro turn and walk away, stepping around the discarded buckets, sandals and clothes, heading back to Confirmed through the scraggly brush, kicking up red dust with their rubber boots.

Dorine and I look at one another, with me feeling obligated to comment. "Boy, if he's gone from here that's going to really suck. Did you hear anything about this in your nurses' tent this morning?"

Dorine shakes her head, answering, "No. And if someone did know they probably were told not to talk about it."

"You really think they would try and keep this quiet?" I asked, somewhat incredulous. "The more people that know and the sooner they know, the better chance we have finding him."

"People do not like to talk about bad things so they stay quiet, hoping it is less bad," Dorine explains, her sincerity genuine.

I stand up erect, exaggerating my looking around the entire ETU, spreading my arms. "Well, if that's the case, they sure sucked at keeping all this secret."

Dorine's two discharges are out the door and down the drive so we turned back to get the other three out of Confirmed. All three are young adult females, maybe 16 to 20 years old. When we go into Confirmed Two, our three patients have the beds closest to the door and closest to the radio, a position that gives them a measure of control over what was being listened to and when. All three are sitting up and lined up, braiding each other's hair and primping. To look at them you'd never think they were sick. I then remembered having treated them earlier on another day, their fondness for one another striking me as something out of the opening scene from Macbeth, though nothing sinister in their nature was present. It is too easy to take the indifference of the ill personally sometimes. The sick are not in the mood for idle conversation, introversion actually being one of the signs of the seriousness of an illness. This morning, all three simply look at me but smile at reading the name 'Dorine' on my partner's apron. All 4 start talking at once and the verbal melee escalates into laughter then when Dorine tells them to get ready to go to the shower.

The Krio conversation goes over my head but finally Dorine includes me, saying, "They do not want a boy to shower them."

I shrug my shoulders, agreeing, "Perfectly fine. I wish them the best." Then looking at all three, not being able to help thinking how much they were like a bunch of high school girls the way they stuck together, I offer a congratulations, saying, "You've made it through something pretty tough. I wish the best for the rest of your lives. Congratulations on being able to go home."

With that, the oldest girl extends the wing of her elbow, inviting me to bump it. We bump and she smiles. "Thank you," then laughs, her eyes wide with mischief, "but I hope to never see you again, Reeck!" pointing at my name. Then all three start repeating my name in unison, having a great time repeating it over and over, laughing all the harder with each repeat. 'So high school', I think to myself, then wave them good-bye and into Dorine's capable hands. "Dorine, I'm going to walk around the grounds and see if there's any sign of that kid."

Outside on the front walk is the usual collection of patients waiting for the worst of the illness or over the worst of the illness. I watch for a moment as the corpse team lifts out a body. Four men each have a hand on a bag handle, the head and foot end drooping towards the ground and the men not compensating for weight by having to lean, cluing me in that it is probably a small woman or child. They come down the walk towards me, clad in pure white, the body bag in white to deliver the deceased into an all white tarped morgue. The moment carries a sense of the transcendent, a step over that invisible line in the universe to another side. I squeeze against the wall to let them pass. They all look through me as they pass, step off the concrete porch and march down to the corner to where the morgue will house the body until the afternoon burial team comes to pick her or him up.

I follow them for a moment then head south to the blue tarped fence, deciding that my search will start at the perimeter of the fence to see if there was possibly any way Mariatu Sesay could have gone under the fence. It's quiet out back, far enough away that one can't hear the constant chatter of workers nor the groans and pleas of patients. Looking off into the distant horizon under an African winter solstice noon sun, the warmth that normally plagues all of us actually feels good. As I look east, it comes to mind that Africa is the Dark Continent, a place so large that it overcomes the visitor with enormous mystery, luring the curious to step into the bush to see what the next 100 yards might reveal, and then the next and so on and so forth, until they are on outskirts of the world's largest desert, the Sahara, or in the thickest imaginable jungles of the Congo. The palm trees in the direction I'm looking get more sparse the further out as they fade into the sub Sahara and away from the more humid and moist coast. In those bushes, I beg for the wish of a lifetime to be fulfilled, to see a cheetah or lion or elephant. I certainly wouldn't object to spying a bushbuck or kob grazing in the out-beyond. A certain resigned sadness comes over me as I realize how much trouble African wildlife in general is in due to human survival pressures that force people to the fringes of damaged economies, force them to take their nutrition from what used to be a cornucopia of plenty no one ever imagined could ever run out. Then again, no one imagined a world with 7 billion people going on 9 billion either. I stand and let it wash over me, praying I can take the good memories to my own end when, I, too, am carried away.

A drizzle of sweat rolls over my eyelid to remind me why I'm out here. A person can curse PPE all they want but they too have admit it makes for great sunscreen.

I walk the fence looking for places where a boy could crawl through to the outside. The top of the fence is over my head and there is no where he could climb out, but along the bottom there is the occasional animal hole dug underneath the tarp, most likely by dogs that come in the middle of the night to scavenge. I reach down to see if I can pick up the bottom of the fence tarp but notice that it is nailed to a bottom stick extended between posts. Mariatu would have to get under the stick, but there are only a couple of inches of room the entire length I inspect. Even the two dog holes I find are small, not large enough to let the shoulders of a boy of 8 years get through, probably not even large enough for his head to fit.

I get to the morgue gate and see that it's open. Peeking out, there is no one around unless you count the four deceased lying on the concrete waiting for burial. Grabbing the latch, I take note of the way it is latched and observe that it is no great security set-up, that anyone from either inside or out could simply slide the bar and walk in or out. Even an 8 year old. But I have my doubts since a person who would leave in this manner would very likely head up the drive and out to the black topped road, then pick a direction of right or left. Would Mariatu wander off into the bush? At night, it was a waning moon in its last quarter, giving him some light. The sulfur solar powered lamps surrounding the ETU and up and down the main road out front would be more inviting. Would he have the presence of mind to consider his leaving something he should hide as best as he could, avoiding the police or other workers out front? Whoever stayed over for night shift most often slept, mainly because it was too troublesome to go back home, meaning Mariatu could have wandered by unnoticed if it were in the early morning hours. Out in town, or on the road, would the community think anything of an 8 year old boy walking alone? I'm pretty certain an 8 year old would know enough to name his village, at least a few relatives, his full name and describe where he came from or is from. I point myself in the direction of the doffing station, thinking he could have very easily walked through to the outside, went down the walkway and out the front gate door to the road. Him going into the bush would only make sense if he viewed his leaving as escape where he needed to hide himself. I could only conclude it was highly unlikely he left with other discharges unnoticed or escaped to the bush by intention, even less so by accident due to the lighting. More likely was the possibility he simply wandered out the morgue gate, discharge gate or through the doffing station gates and did so during light hours, walking through the day crowd, just another child belonging to one of the workers, no one even noticing the patient wrist band. Yet, out in the Port Loko town area, an 8 year old would eventually have to petition for help in getting home, revealing himself, tagged by his plastic wristband that he could not remove by himself.

There's a line at doffing so rather than wait around, I decide to head to the hot zone side towards the worker shower area outside a few steps from the doffing station, a place where there is no restriction between the hot zone and green zone oddly enough, the only deterrent being that it is relatively obscure to find, but not impossible to find if you wander about for a few minutes on the grounds. Here the fire pit was smoldering away, the contaminated PPE's, blankets, lafas and all manner of burnable refuse imaginable. The smell reminds me of my childhood growing up down the road from a public dump where garbage was always being set fire, smoke creeping out over my small town to leave malodorous hints of its existence. Stinky, yes, but a source of great entertainment for kids who like to shoot rats, cans or bottles with BB gun and watch fires. I walk in closer to the pit, overhung with a tin roof on thick sticks, cinder block stacked and masoned three blocks deep rising off the ground for its perimeter. Grabbing one of the stick rails on the end away from where smoke is rising, looking down I see that the pit itself is a good ten feet deep and that there is a wooden hand built ladder that only a fool would step onto, especially since wooden ladders in fire pits are not symbiotic unless you consider the wood of the ladder an appropriate addition of fuel to the fire. The acridity of the smoke stings my eyes and even when it clears away from me, I'm unable to see well enough to the bottom, my visor being scratched and dull not helping. Already today the cleaning crews have been through the grounds and dumped their hauls, which is usually about six 35 gallon trash cans worth by best guestimate. That would be enough to cover up quite a few things.

A second fire pit is being built nearby about 10 yards away, with the hole dug and cinder blocks in place waiting for its tin roof. Peering down there is nothing but dirt, waiting for its first use burn. I go back to the first fire pit and see one of the cleaners hauling a black plastic trash bag with him and then throwing it into the pit.

"Hey," I shout to get his attention. He turns around and I see the name Racin written across his apron. As he gets closer to me, he sees my name and gives me his usual enthusiastic greeting, "Reeck! What you do here, man?" giving me his extended elbow to bump.

"Got a question for you," I start off, "how often they dump and burn in this pit?"

Racin looks at the pit then back at me, shrugging, "Pretty much once a day in the mornings. The fire never really goes out."

"The fire doesn't burn out so it doesn't have to be relit. You can just keep adding garbage?" I ask.

Racin nods. "Pretty much, now that it is dry season. By the end of the day there's not much smoke, but sometimes the fire will start up again depending how wet the garbage is."

"Does it get a good flame?" I ask. "You know, one that would be sort of fun to watch?"

Racin looks at me through his equally scarred visor, pausing before he speaks. "Oh, sure. Sometimes it takes off enough and gets high enough to char the wood," pointing at the haphazard stick railings set up around the pit, blackened by smoke and heat. "Sometimes it even gets high enough to see over the sides."

I think about this and what I'm thinking isn't good. Is this something we need to consider? Would Mariatu be curious enough to come back to this fire pit and poke around, maybe even lean over the side to watch the fire, silly enough to try to walk the perimeter cinder blocks, assuming the smoke and smell were at a tolerable ebb. A certain amount of substitution on my part was taking place, referencing my own childhood fascination with fire where my friends and I would burn our model cars in horrific, imaginary crashes. Maybe we'd find some old refrigerator box, or a car fender shipping box my dad would bring home from the shop for us to demolish, though our burning it was not on his syllabus. Fire fascinates many children. Why not Mariatu?

I break off my thought, turning back to my fellow Ebola fighter, saying, "Thanks, Racin."

"Why you so curious about this fire pit?" Racin asks.

"You don't want to know," shaking my head. "Let's go eat."

As we walk towards the doffing station, Racin asks me to explain my questions. I tell him the story of the missing 8 year old boy but that he most likely he wandered off through one of the several ways out, unnoticed.

Racin listens intently, then follows my story with information of rumors, telling me that he heard something about looking for an eight year old. I ask him if he heard if they were looking in town, trying to find family, whatever. Racin professed to know no details, just that he heard about trying to find some lost 8 year old, not even knowing if the child was a patient.

We both get to the doffing station and spread eagle to start the doffing process. Racin looks at me and shakes his head, saying, "Do we even want to look," nodding towards the pit. "I know I wouldn't want to know."

In my own thoughts, I'm thinking of how to get into the pit to look without risking a hazard. It would take some planning. Racin's speaking brings me out to consider what he said and I reply, "You might be right. Maybe we don't want to know."

With that we focus on our doffing, trying to stay out of the way of the carpenters trying to expand the doffing station. Hammers, nails, tin sheeting are scattered over the doffing area, requiring an added piece of attention not to trip or slice one's self.

For the afternoon, I end up shifted over to the admissions building to help walk in the new admissions, staying busy due to ambulances lined up waiting turns to divulge their human cargo. Jabari had the foresight to recruit two national nurses to help us out so we could run staggered teams. No sooner than we would get one or two patients from one ambulance settled than there was another at the ready, forcing us to rotate through, meaning that as soon as one task was done, we would doff, walk back over to the admissions building, take a good drink and don again to tend the next set of patients.

The afternoon rolls by, another record pace for admissions, indicating that the crisis is not waning here in Sierra Leone like it has in Liberia. Finally it's time to call it a day. Ibrahim is waiting outside the gate in his green Dodge minivan. Musa and me are the last two to go home with him heading to the Dutch camp and then me to the Ghetto. During our chat, just when Musa is starting to tell me how he ended up getting a college football scholarship, he stops talking, his eyes focused out the side window.

"Stop the car!" Musa shouts.

Ibrahim stomps on the brakes, hard enough my seat belt locks me in. Musa throws open the door, shouting, "That's the kid."

I follow Musa out the door, looking to see what he's seeing, and spot a boy, about 8, running away from us. For a big man, Musa's motor is running and I have to pour it on to catch up. Both of us are gaining on the boy as he runs smack down the middle of the pavement, oncoming traffic ignoring our chase and giving us wide berth. As the boy runs, he turns to look at us and see how close we're getting, the expression on his face one of sheer terror, boosting his adrenaline probably a bit more to quicken his pace. Thirty feet behind him now and closing, the boy takes a left turn off the road and onto the red gravel, running up to a mud brick house where he stops on the porch and hides behind a man who is now watching us, wondering what terrible thing we might be doing. At this, Musa pulls up and stops, catching his breath then raising his hands, shouting to the boy and the man, "Sorry. Wrong person. We thought it was someone else."

Both of us stay put as the man comes off his porch and walks towards us, confident in his stride. We wait. I can only imagine that he's going to express his displeasure in angry terms but find just the opposite as Musa engages the fellow in Krio, explaining the story of our missing

Mariatu Sesay and the mistaken identity. Fortunately for us, the man who is the father of the boy we just chased, understands and seems to express his sympathy and accepts Musa's apology, bidding us 'Shalom' as we leave.

Ibrahim followed us the quarter mile down the road, the side door open, laughing at how a big man like Musa could move so fast. We drop Musa at Dutch camp then Ibrahim and I go through town via city circle, now filled with people out for evening walks, catching up with their neighbors. At a local water hole, Ibrahim and I stop for cold beers and sodas at one of the two places I know that has a working freezer and head back to the Ghetto.

Supper is already out on the table so I hurry through my bucket bath, having learned that standing in the bucket is one of the better ways to clean up and catch the dirty water to keep it from spilling all over the bathroom. Outside my door, shorts, socks and underwear I put out from the night before to have washed are neatly folded and ready for me to change into for the evening.

At supper, we discuss the day's work, the missing child and the expansion of the schedule into evening hours and, eventually, night shift hours, for staffing the ETU when more arrivals land in the next couple of weeks. As night falls, Tigger lies on the sand pile, sated from the various left over fish and other table scraps put down for him. The crescent of a waning moon is high enough that we can see it over the compound's glass studded walls, silvery blue with a tinge of red from the dust in the air. Several people wander out the gate and down to the big tree to go talk with Bernard, the local who is the head of the burial team for the Port Loko district. There, he and some friends and family chat away the dark, sipping whiskey gifted by Doc Peterson a couple of days ago. David invites me to meet Bernard, an older fellow by Sierra Leone standards and about David's age. We pass time, getting local updates, educated on local customs and speculate on the whereabouts of Mariatu. Then we leave, feeling the whiskey, both of us wondering if the kid sees the same moon.

Black Jacket

The arrival of new clinicians continues, each with a resume more impressive than the next. Specialists ranging from advanced nurse practitioners, infectious disease experts and emergency room doctors were the norm, but in getting to know their backgrounds, it was their other passions in life that made them unique. Todd, an RN, was an ultra marathoner, having competed in more than a few 100 mile plus races. Then there was Jim the RN who doubled as a clown, using his show business talent to entertain pediatric patients. He also belonged to an international organization that promoted the same, Clowns Without Borders. Others like Betty, Mary and Lawrence had backgrounds that they overcame which lent them an empathy you cannot fake. In the medical setting, that empathy, or lack of it, is summed up under the title of bedside manner. I thought when I became a nurse that I had it, learning later, the hard way, that maybe I didn't as much as I would have liked.

In 2004, I became ill, noticing the first symptoms after a dinner of salmon, asparagus, salad and white wine made for me by a friend at her home on Case Inlet, near Olympia, Washington. There, I worked at one of the local hospitals. What I thought was simple indigestion worsened to the point I could not or did not want to eat, attempting to avoid spikes in abdominal pain that came with a meal. Previous to all this, I had been diagnosed with ulcerative colitis and took a daily medication to keep it under control, something that worked so well that I never even gave it a second thought that I was dealing with a chronic disease.

Days ticked by and I worked, but with great discomfort. Normally, I exercised regularly, ran a couple of marathons a year or swam to stay in shape and pass the time, never weighing less than 150 pounds on my 5'9" frame. During those sick days that crawled by, pound after pound started to drop, with the pain so intense that in one 12 day period I made 8 emergency room visits, hoping find out what was going on and receive badly needed pain relief. Each visit was perfunctory and routine in the manner that I would relate my past health history, exercise routine, current status of pain and rapid weight loss. Each time, the ER doc would claim it was my exercise routine causing the weight loss, an absurd diagnosis in light of the incredible pain I was having and that the illness halted my normal daily routine in its tracks. When I expressed a desire for opiate pain relief, something that in the previous 7 visits provided instant relief and literally gave me a life free of the physically and spiritually crushing pain, pain that had me fetal when I wasn't working, the ER doc decided I was drug seeking and that he saw no reason to call in the GI specialist.

Of course, I tried to get in to see my own GI doc but he was booked out 3 weeks in advance. Knowing this, I pleaded with the ER doc to call in my doc who happened to be on call the eighth time I was in the ER. He relented. An hour later, a quick sigmoidoscopy showed on the exam screen a colon that was completely ulcerated, a real mess that even a layman could ID as not healthy tissue. Unfortunately, my GI doc was unable to pinpoint the cause of all the pain, as ulcerative colitis is generally not so painful. When it is, opiates are used with great caution since they can slow down the normal motility of the GI tract, leading to a buildup of life threatening toxins. So, no more pain control.

Two more weeks passed and, finally, 30 days and 30 pounds lighter, I took vacation time, got on a plane and flew back to Wisconsin, hoping prescribed steroids and antibiotics would finally help. After 5 days of lying around my parents, scaring them half to death with my sickly look, I ended up in my hometown ER where the doc did something I still kick myself for not thinking of earlier: he pulled an amylase-lipase blood test to check for pancreatitis. Bingo. Cause of pain diagnosed.

I was admitted in hopes of healing my colon and controlling the pancreatic pain. The later was well controlled with an opiate pain pump, but the former, my colon, failed to respond to treatment so under the knife I went, waking up with an ostomy on my belly exactly as my father did at the same age. For the next seven months, there were three more surgeries, CT scans galore, parenteral nutrition by IV, infections, night sweats, tamponade of the left lung requiring needle aspiration, pancreatic stent placements, gall bladder removal and me relearning to eat.

Every day, medical people were in and out of my room and I would ask to know what my latest test results showed and, to my utter surprise, the majority simply refused to discuss them, leaving the room as if I never asked the question. Most nurses would come in and change my IV bags and avoid my attempts at casual conversation, let alone answer any questions I had on the latest scan or lab draw. This struck me as odd at first and I blamed myself for somehow offending them, but it became clear that they didn't know the answers, that taking the time to learn my chart was not a priority. It wasn't until my 7th month, after I was shipped back out to Seattle at my insurance company's demands, did a nurse and my surgeon, on the final hospitalization to perform the takedown surgery to remove the temporary ostomy, actually spend time to discuss what I had been through and what I should expect going forward. I was not at all prepared for the emotional impact the simple act of wanting to know about me, and how I was coping, rather than just my disease, would have on me. Separate of one another, they ordered a visiting pet come to see me, the hospital golden retriever that actually was happy enough he put his front paws up on my bed to lick my face and let me scruff him about the neck to play wrestle. It left a profound impression about how to look at, and how to engage, the person on their back. Patients want to know how their disease works, how they can cope with it, what may or may not work and why.

When I took this new perspective back onto the hospital floor after I became well again, I tested it by asking patients if they knew what their diagnoses was, if they knew why they were admitted. I was astonished to find that about 3 out of 4 patients could not give layman terms for their admission, let alone what their possible treatment plan was or its likelihood of success or failure. You can't know what someone fails to teach. Since that time, I still ask those two questions: Can you tell me why or what you're here for in the hospital, and, do you know what the plan is to fix it. By the way, you have any allergies to dogs?

Patients are in a vulnerable position, rendering many to be passive, mostly out of not knowing where to start asking questions. There is always the take-charge patient who pushes to know, who won't leave you alone until they are satisfied their questions have been answered to the best of your ability. Moreover, when they aren't satisfied with your best, go beyond you to wherever it is they will find what it is they seek. They are a distinct minority, so much so that they are often memorable.

So, here in Port Loko, for all of the collective talent and all the dedication, I was acutely aware of our limits in communicating with our patients. Make no mistake, the greatest expression of empathy towards a patient is the acquisition of skill to fix their ailment. Flowers and candy are generous and wonderful, but patients need hands that touch to heal as well as to console. One we focus on with great effort to learn, the other we just think we know.

On the morning walks to work, I found it fun to watch the nurses and docs I worked with engage the locals. At no time did anyone ever try to take advantage of their own position over that of the locals. Haggling was expected in the majority of dealings with merchants and every person in the organization did so, but everyone also pulled their punches, so to speak, to not take advantage of their relative wealth in contrast to that of the local mother cooking dough to make morning doughnuts or the carpenter assembling, by hand, our medicine chests.

These small acts were observable on the walks in other ways, such as dealing with the myriad of dogs that had a look they all descended from the same two or three breeds. Even after Keri's disconcerting encounter with the dog that chomped into her backpack, she continued buying her doughnuts and continued to pick out one or two dogs to share her snacking breakfast. The others would try to name a favorite dog, but out of the literally hundreds one could see in a typical walk, and the fact that they were so similar, it was pretty much impossible to remember a given dog.

Tigger would follow us from the compound for about a half-mile before peeling off and heading back to his sand pile at the Ghetto. When he did, the other dogs would get tight on our heels, hoping for that snack or the consolation prize of a pat on the head. Some might call this petting of strange animals something on the foolhardy side in light of the risk of rabies, a very real problem where veterinary care, especially preventive care like distemper or rabies vaccines, simply was nonexistent. But they would be petted, lovingly mocked, praised or simply allowed to tag along until we reached the Bankasoka bridge, neither a boundary the town dogs seemed to want to cross nor the country dogs, either. Some mornings, as many as 50 dogs would stop at the bridge to watch us walk off into the distance. The dogs would then turn back, heading up the hill into town.

On this morning walk, Bernard passed us in the Red Cross/Red Crescent body truck, honking as he passed, most likely out to arrange for new gravesites and to tally how much work lay ahead for the burial teams he was overseeing. Down on the riverbank was the other RC/RC truck. Ten year old boys were washing it out with water drawn up in buckets from the river, revealing to me for the first time that there were two trucks. More unnerving, was that 10 year old kids were washing these death trucks without any protective gear, unwise, even though the bed of the truck was thoroughly sprayed with disinfectant.

Morning report was the same, just a lot more of it, as increasing numbers of patients arrived. What stuck out this morning was a family of five that came in: a mother with her three children along with the mother's brother. The family of Josephine Kargbo was known to have cared for family members who died from Ebola, and now their kindness was being repaid with the punishment of disease. By all accounts, from their admission intake history taken the day before, each one of them was likely positive and presented with wet symptoms, the only thing holding them out of Confirmed being the pending test results. From the admissions building doorway overlooking the Suspect courtyard, I could see Josephine Kargbo in her black suit jacket, dark navy dress and gray shades of her head wrap. It was as if she dressed to express her mourning. All three children, ages 3, 5 and 7, were sitting next to her with not a hint of any smile. Josephine's brother appeared absent.

We picked up our assignments; I was assigned a national and a new arrival doctor, Betty, a Montana ER doctor, to care for the patients in C-3 and C-4. After only two days, Dr. Betty had it down pat on what supplies to gather up, how to prepare them prior to entry and in general plan ahead for any contingencies. A small team like ours made communication and decision making much easier since her MD degree became the natural terminal of the final say, a hierarchy that we were comfortable with. When one is teamed with equals, the tendency is to grant equal legitimacy to one another's ideas and stalemates can develop that are nothing more than time killers. More is done with a minute of leadership than an hour of debate.

Inside, we made quick work going bed to bed, recharging spent IV's, administering antimalaria drugs and antibiotics per the bedside charts, and assessing signs and symptoms to track improvements and declines. Patients in wet clothes were stripped, washed down and given dry garments, usually a lafa, and maybe some Valium by mouth or syringe. Paracetamol was given to ease whatever discomforts they had, even though Valium and Paracetamol are poor substitutes as pain control products, but that being the best allowed for reasons that were infuriating, condescending and patronizing.

I'm convinced that the International Narcotics Control Board, overseen by the United Nations, was configured to provide a job for someone's out of place brother-in-law. Under the guise of the War on Drugs, there is the attitude that third world nations are not capable of managing opiate painkillers. In the midst of a tragic crisis, it upset me to no end hearing of higher-ups, staying at Freetown hotels, stuffing their faces with fresh seafood served buffet style in mounds, rationalizing to one another how it was not worth the effort to pipeline in some real painkillers for those in the worst throes of the disease. The very reason for the existence of medicine is to eradicate physical, psychological or spiritual discomfort. A significant part of the problems our patients were having was their wrenched guts, bones that felt as if they had pipe wrenches cranking away at them. On top of that, there was the skull crushing headaches and full body muscle pain as capillaries ruptured and red blood cells exploded, contributing to massive fluid displacements that put pressure on sensitive parts of the body behind the eyes, eardrum and joint spaces. If you ever want to find how much of a nobody you are, notice a problem then find out how powerless you are to fix it even when you have the knowledge of how it should be fixed. By that standard, I'm a pretty big nobody but, even worse, my patients appeared to be even bigger nobodies.

Our round went well. No bodies needed removing, though the corpse team was occupied removing two others from C-1 or C-2. With some time to spare, Dr. Betty decided that we could stay and rehang additional IV fluids rather than waiting for the afternoon round, a perfectly good idea, and a chance to help the patients catch up on their fluid losses from overnight.

As we rehung the last of the second round of IV bags, outside at the gate separating Suspect from Confirmed, two white suits shouted at me and Betty that they had the Kargbo family ready to be admitted into Confirmed. Betty and I went to the gate and could see it was Jim, the clown fellow, and Susy, another new arrival nurse, both who blessed us with the good fortune of being badly needed pediatric nurses.

"Who do we have here?" Betty asked.

Jim held up his list and read out loud, "Well, they are the Kargbo family. All six of them. All came back positive and they asked us to move them over here. That's OK, right?"

Dr. Betty looked over the clan, all carrying buckets, but a couple of the children a bit wobbly and all twelve eyes bloodshot. But no hiccups. "Oh, yes, we have time to settle them if you have other things to do."

"We do," Jim apologetically offered, explaining, "there are a couple of kids we haven't seen yet. We just wanted to get this family over here before everyone was done."

Susy apologized on their behalf again, saying, "We would do it but we just are running out of time."

Dr. Betty graciously absolved Jim and Susy by expressing her understanding and reassuring them it was no problem at all.

But I did have a problem. "You mentioned that this was the whole Kargbo family. I thought there were only five if I recall report correctly. Who is the sixth one?" As I looked over the crew, I easily accounted for all five by being able to read their wristbands. Before I could ascertain the name on the sixth person, Jim gave me the names on his list and finished with, "...and the last is Sally Kargbo."

"15 years old?" I asked.

"Yes. How'd you know that?" Jim asked.

Crap. "Sally isn't part of this family. She just shares the same last name.

At least I think she isn't part of this family."

Dr. Betty picked up on all this quickly and waved Sally towards her and closer to the gate, asking, "Sally, I'm Dr. Betty. Are you part of this family?"

Sally lifted her eyes from the ground, searching through our visors for some hint of humanity, then saying, in an almost whisper, "No, I am alone. We just share the last name."

With that, I jump in and explain that Sally was here at the ETU about 10 days back and put into Suspect for having a fever, but eventually had a PCR that came back negative and was discharged to home.

Betty looks at me, letting the impact of that information seep in, and then saying, "Oh, no, do you think she wasn't infected but became infected here?"

I shrug. "Maybe. Likely."

"And you're not part of this family, Sally?" Dr. Betty gently inquired again.

Before she can answer, Josephine reaches back and grabs Sally by the wrist, pulling her up to the front of the queue, next to her. In as firm of a voice as a healthy person could muster, let alone a sick one, Josephine, with emphasis, disagrees, saying, "No. She is now part of our family. She will stay with us." Then she stares all four of us down, daring us to object. The uncle moves in closer to show his solidarity and the three children sense the rally and vote by huddling in closer to their new 'aunt' or 'big sister'.

None of us had any objections--or any reason to object. If that right belonged to anyone, it was the five natural Kargbo's who had it, but instead they chose to bring in the stranger. Maybe it was the coincidental last name or maybe it was just understanding that no one should be left alone. It is so easy to forget that when you are sick that others still have needs and wants. Hell, it's hard enough to realize that when you are well and healthy, going day to day about one's own routine, to remember how it impacts others.

With that, Betty opens the gate to let the clan through.

watching, not comfortable with the entire situation.

"I'm not giving you anything, Right now, what I see is four men out of gear, violating strict body handling protocol." Then I pulled my trump card, continuing, "What do you think Bernard would think of this."

My confronter's face froze. I continued, piling it on, saying, "You're out of gear. Could lose your job over this if I choose to report it to Bernard, and then I'd have to tell him about the torn body bag and the two dogs that came running out from an unlocked morgue. That's how the dogs got in, right? Someone, probably you, hasn't been locking the morgue?"

"We lock each time," he replied, shuffling his feet, continuing, "and it is the corpse teams who fail the lock."

"No, I doubt that. The corpse team enters through the side door from the ETU and cannot exit the loading dock," I explained. "If you try that side door, you won't be able to open it from inside the morgue. It's bolted from inside the ETU. If you look, you can see the pin in it now. No one from this side is going go through that door unless someone opens it for them from the ETU side."

Turning on his heels and walking away from me, I had a quick idea. "If you and you're work mates give me a picture, Bernard doesn't find out about this."

He pauses at the rear of the cab, soaking his hands in bleach spray, replying, "OK. One photo."

With that compromise, all four gathered in while I focused and snapped my one allowed photo. The three others beamed with bright smiles and asked to look at the digital record, pleased as punch. The man with the frown was having issues with me.

"One more thing," trying my best to give him back his leadership role, I asked,, "Would it ever be possible to see the cemetery? Bernard said it would be OK but I think asking you when makes more sense."

The man shook his head in exasperated disbelief as he wiggled out of his PPE, then spoke, saying, "Go in the evening. After 5. All day there are funerals. Do not disturb the mourners if they are there. And, please, no photos."

"Certainly. No pictures. Perfectly understandable. Thank you," I said, doing my best to be gracious. "You have to promise me something: you will put on your hoods and masks every time. I know the body bags are sprayed down and pose a low risk but it is still a real risk." Then pointing to the ETU, I continue, "This place is not a good place to end up in. It is about the worst thing I can imagine happening to someone. You really never want to be like any of these people inside. So, promise me you guys, full dress from now on."

All four nodded in agreement, seeming comfortable and trusting that I wouldn't rat them out to Bernard. Burial team members earned a wage of about 500,000 Leones a week, a veritable fortune in a country with unemployment running near 80% in the Port Loko district. The loss of their jobs would bring back hardship they were risking their lives to avoid, clinging to an economic cliff to keep from falling into the poverty abyss.

I watched three of them load into the cab of the truck while the odd man out hopped into the rear bed, in full gear, and took a seat on one of the bodies. Off they went, delivering the end result of our failure to heal. As I walked back up the drive to head back for the afternoon round, behind me in the ETU, minister birds were cackling over morsels of left out food, scavenging the garbage and spillage, a golden opportunity, enjoying the fringe benefits of our sad operation. Two birds were chasing one who had a thumb-sized piece of bread, trying to force him to drop it. If they succeeded, it certainly wasn't like the two aggressors would split the loot, but instead make the loser an ally of the bird left out of his share of the treasure. Funny how animals are so much like people, I thought.
■■■

Lockdown

The Ghetto dinner hour was the routine that relieved and refreshed with meals of chicken, fish, potatoes, salad fixings and local fruits and vegetables. Tomatoes were at every dinner for salad and there was a rumor that wild tomatoes were growing behind the morgue, something I wanted to see, and if any way possible, see if I could get the seeds back to the States and try growing them. Of course taking something from inside the ETU to the outside is about as sacrosanct of rule there is, making it imperative that I find a way to disinfect the tomatoes, package them and then get them outside without incident. It wasn't consuming me to complete this plot but it was as good as a distraction as our supper hour as we shared stories and learned more about each other.

Our one Christmas decoration, a banner spelling out 'Merry Christmas' hung between the patio rafters, evidence of someone's forward thinking that they packed it into their luggage. In a country 80-85% Muslim, Christmas isn't exactly a priority holiday, but the Sierra Leone Muslims did participate in the traditions, gatherings and meals along with their Christian counterparts, the sectarian violence further inland perpetrated by Boko Haram and other violent religious groups, rejected by the West African nations as an immoral perversion of faith. Too many people were in the prime of their lives with memories of the political civil war 15 years earlier, understanding firsthand the destruction and backwardness of conflicts. A conflict premised on differing faiths, something far more philosophically entrenched in peoples' lives, would be an insanity bringing the possible chronic nightmare of acts of genocide.

Christmas Eve dinner was scheduled outside the Ghetto at a nightclub down the road, everyone from the all the various aid organizations invited for a big night of food and drink and a chance to blow off some steam. No one had a day off yet that I was aware of and soon the evening and night shifts would be starting up, throwing away the healthy luxury of day shifts and being able to sleep in fan cooled rooms at night since, during the day, the generator was idle. On good source, we heard the Mansion and Sugar Shack, a defunct disco nightclub turned into a boarding house, pink, blue and bright green, where many new arrivals were being put up, had showers and all day electricity. Not one person from the Ghetto ever complained. Complaining would only make matters worse, that being any solution would result in someone being displaced from a comfortable place to a place that had...well, certain challenges like bucket showers and no air conditioning. Who wants to be the person that bellyaches about their accommodations and then gets someone tossed to make room for someone else's upgrade? It would be a pretty callous person and, with healthcare workers, it would be less apt to occur then say maybe Wall Street traders. Moreover, we had pet geckos, bats, dog on a pile of sand and a nightclub a five minute walk distant. The poor Sugar Shack was across from a prison and The Mansion was on the outskirts of town, not within walking distance of local markets. Location, location, location.

But our location and the holidays came with a caveat, that being the country was put on lockdown for 3 days with no movement in or out of the villages, towns and districts, all commercial traffic halted plus no celebratory gatherings.

On our list, we were told to pack a set of decent clothes for trips or gatherings to the US embassy, which was about as likely to happen as me meeting Neil Armstrong. The Christmas Party was as good as an opportunity to get into some nice clothes as I was going to have, something to look forward to as much as a holiday video chat with family back in Ohio and Wisconsin. The latter failed, with the internet apparently on lockdown as well, our connection so poor that the only merciful thing to do was euthanize and go off-line. The former, the party, was an incredible meal of meats, casseroles, fresh fruits and vegetables, along with liquor, wine and beer and a women's arm wrestling match cooked up by Patti and Francie with those two facing off against each other.

Patti had youth and college basketball experience on her side while Francie had attitude and the experience of age. For weeks Francie had been talking up the competition and the Christmas party was also the last day of her assignment, making it the logical venue for a crowd and as good as diversion as we were going to get. The two took seats at the end of one of the banquet tables, locked hands and started on a referee's signal. Francie lasted for a good while but athletic youth held the upper hand, giving the olive wreath to Patti. As far as I was concerned, we as a group collectively lost by losing Francie and the other members of the Frontier Four.

I have no idea why our party wasn't affected by the lockdown and our venue was allowed to stay open to host the shindig. Idle speculation was that the suitcase of Leones one of the logicians rolled around for emergencies found an emergency. On the other hand, there was the locked metal gate with its door that was open when the establishment was open but was now closed, requiring a knock where a person on the other side would size us up looking through a slide trap then let us in like some sort of 1920's Chicago speakeasy. Rules work when they are good ideas and the lockdown was a fine idea, but the Christmas party was a better idea.

We all had our fill and busted out before midnight to head back to our compounds, having work the next morning. The walk back was in near pitch black with only a fingernail sliver of the new moon. Further down the road, a seasonal brush fire was burning away the last season's undergrowth, casting a helpful but smoky light, aggravating the chlorine cough Adam and a couple of others had developed and still hadn't shaken. All the homes were dark. Even the residents one might see sitting out late to look out over the neighborhood were indoors. It was as if someone flipped a switch and turned off the entire town.

I expected a quiet breakfast but soon realized that we were all in the same routine; the same morning chatter went on. Most decided to walk. Early along the route, where we met up with the markets, this morning there were only snoozing dogs and the usual goats we'd see were absent. No smell of cooking fires and no one in the commercial stalls. No motorcycles or trucks beeping away or the normal knot of motorcycle taxis in the city center circle waiting for dispatch. No pedestrians hauling wood, bundles of palm, oranges or bananas. I expected to hear a child shouting 'Apatow' but even that was missing. The switch was turned off. In a country where millions live an existence hand to mouth, the lockdown was strangling their ability to feed themselves, the order coming with only several days notice. Liberia attempted the same strategy and in hindsight, even the president who ordered it, considered it a poor idea and a failure, the lesson not rubbing off on its neighbor.

Of the few people out in the morning, I recognized only one, an Imam of a beautiful mosque maybe a century old next to the incomplete hydroelectric project, the thing which was supposed to make all switches work having its own switch indefinitely off. Each morning on our walk, the Imam would be out in his front yard, on the red gravel pacing leisurely with an open copy of the Quran, stopping to read then resuming his comfortable pacing. On several mornings, he came up near the road, letting us be the ones to stop and talk rather than the other way around. His English was halting, but understandable, as we exchanged pleasantries and minor personal information, only revealing his Imam status when someone inquired. The attire should have been enough to announce his calling. This morning, dressed in a white and gold robe and matching skullcap, he waited for us by the roadside, raising his hand for our attention. Major Dennis and Adam were in the lead and the first to stop, the rest of us falling into the group. With his Quran open, the large rainy season concrete gutter separating our group from him, about 5 feet apart, he motioned us in as close as possible and read a short time from the Quran in what sounded like Krio.

On Christmas morning, the Imam calculated that maybe we would appreciate a blessing of some sort and his Quran recitation was it, a magnanimous gesture that in some parts of the United States would be mocked, possibly even violently rejected due to the ongoing struggles with terrorism since 9/11. None of us understood what was said but Adam asked to look at the passage, taking a note of the passage numbers. We thanked him for his kindness and Dennis, the most openly Christian amongst us who would also be a guest later that day on a Christian radio show, wished the Imam a hearty Merry Christmas that the Imam took in good grace.

The routine at the ETU was all the same: J Edgar and the guards listening to morning news reports, workers getting on with their jobs, morning prayers in the ETU mosque by some, Ali managing the temperature queue, admonishing us to wash, a rhetorical admonishment since it was all so embedded and automatic in everyone, plus, the local nurses carrying on in good spirits.

Inside the admissions' building, the whiteboard was filled in with the names of yesterday's admissions. Gwyn and her group were filling out the last of the patient information cards for us to copy. Total patient census was now at its highest since Maforki opened back in early November, the graph lines plotting the numbers continued a steady uphill climb. Even though the outlying CCC's that Adam, Dr. Peterson, Patti and Chris helped establish were now taking some patients, the workload was continuing to become more intense. The District Emergency Reports Census, issued daily, was not a source of inspiration with all its numbers on new cases, burials, open graves available, admissions, discharges and deaths.

On the walk back to the nurses' station, George was on a bench, resting and not looking very happy. His green eyes and lighter complexion always made him stand out from his co-workers, but his normally gregarious demeanor was missing.

"Morning, George. Merry Christmas," offering my holiday greeting.

Breaking his concentration, George Washington, the name I gave him to help me remember, met me with a forced smile and matched my greeting. "Merry Christmas."

Hesitating to probe any more, we remained in silence until I decided to break the conversational impasse, asking, "No power salute this morning? Are you taking the day off for Christmas?"

Perking up some, George laughed. "No. No day off ever here. We were supposed to have a sprayer's meeting this afternoon with Dr. George to talk about days off and pay. But no more. The Chief of Police came in to tell us that any meeting would be an illegal gathering."

I wasn't following. "How would it be an illegal gathering?"

George gave me a look relaying I must be a bit dense, his voice stressing what should have been obvious to me. "Lockdown. No meetings or gatherings during lockdown."

"I'm sorry to hear that," I said, knowing there were problems. "Are you able to get another meeting set up?"

"He will not reply," George replied, waving his hand in disgust. "This is the third time that he has not shown."

"What do you need help with?" I asked, trying to get specific information.

"We're never sure when we're going to get paid. Some get paid every week. Some haven't been paid in 4 weeks. Our wages are not enough to get along on and they aren't the same every week. One week I got 200,000. The next, I didn't get paid. When I did, the week after it was 200,000 and I was told it was for the last two weeks. My wages dropped by half!" George continued, growing more exasperated as he spoke. "Millions have been promised to help us fight. Where is it? I don't know where it is. Somebody has it, not us."

George was furious. I was helpless. Sympathy is a useless emotion when you can't offer any viable solutions. Even when others claim to stand with someone experiencing problems, without actual help, they stand alone. That is exactly how some people in the world of work would like it to be—for each man to stand alone.

Trying to let George know I cared, I continued engaging him, asking, "You have any ideas at all what you can do?"

"Yes. I know exactly what we will do today," George replied with certainty.

My best guess was George and several others would try to force a meeting with whoever was standing in for Dr. George, or maybe just have a meeting around lunchtime to lay out a plan for when lockdown ended. George was a decent person not given to becoming too excited or worked up over things, able to discern the nuances of the world in a way that some would say made him wise beyond his years. He handled the crews well, never leaving us to wait at doffing despite how irregular we came in or out, always ready at the drop of a hat.

"It seems like you have things under control. Patience is good. Thinking ahead, covering all possibilities, is better," I said, trying to be encouraging.

"Thank you." George got up off the bench and headed inside.

I knelt down to fumble around in my pack for notes to see what I might need from pharmacy. As I was doing this, J Edgar came up behind me, loudly announcing, "Good morning, Reeck. How goes it?"

I turned to see J Edgar in a black sweater over his usual police uniform navy blue short sleeves. "Good. Merry Christmas."

"Merry Christmas to you, too," J Edgar replied. He then leaned into me, lowering his voice so his own officers sitting nearby would not hear him, saying, "There is a rumor that the sprayers will strike today. I have heard they have complaints. If you see signs of trouble, get your distance just to be on the safe side. Go to the admission building or across the road and count everyone in your work group."

I looked at J Edgar, wondering how serious he was. At no time did he ever feel a need to warn us but, then again, there was nothing to warn about. Somehow, he felt this was different, forcing me to ask, "Are you really worried something could happen today?"

J Edgar shrugged, saying, "I don't think so. George is a good person. He doesn't want problems. There are others who might not be so patient anymore. The grumbling is more open now. It will all get fixed in good time but you are not in any danger. If they meet today as a worker's group, it will be illegal because of the lockdown rules. I will have to break it up. That's when I will be worried."

"I'll keep my eyes and ears open," I replied. "But not anything to really worry about, though, right?"

"Absolutely," J Edgar assured me. "Others know. We just don't want the militia involved with anything here. If a lockdown violation happens, they have the right to get involved. We don't want them to have an excuse to do that. Don't worry; you'll be safe."

"Thanks, J Edgar. Appreciate the heads up," I said. "Be careful."

J Edgar flashed a smile and headed back down to his radio and spot in the shade. Complaints by staff anywhere are just part of the job. Most of it is misinformation based on incomplete information and gossip, the predicted disasters never coming to pass. Morning round was going to be busy with the high patient census, so the better prepared I was, the smoother it would go.

The whiteboard showed Dr. Dahna and I paired with two Cubans, Dr. Carlos and Nurse Alonzo and national nurse, Dorine. Dr. Dahna was a recent arrival and this was our first time together. The doctor's recent arrival, along with the Spanish-English dynamic, was going to slow us down unless we split our patients.

At the pharmacy, Dr. Dahna was a step ahead of me, going down her list of protocol medications, bagging what she expected to need. Together, we finished up our morning gathering and headed back to the nurses' station to start drawing up the Artesimin, Rocephin and Flagyl, sorting out the various IV antibiotics, syringes and other meds that usually needed restocking . Her systematic preparations lent confidence to our upcoming round. The kicker was, she knew some Spanish. As lead, she decided that keeping us in one group was the better idea, which made sense since she would be able to talk with Dr. Carlos.

I gathered Dr. Carlos, Alonzo and Dorine. The five of us finished our donning and headed in, red bio bags in hand along with water, rags and a couple of blankets for the cooler nights. I remember thinking to myself how funny it would be if we were inside and all the sprayers went on strike, leaving us stranded to doff on our own. Whatever their motivations, their unhappiness had nothing to do with us, though I wondered how they would have felt if they knew what us expats were being compensated. As for what Alonzo and Carlos were being paid, that was a complete mystery. Cuba is a poor country and displays of wealth are considered bad form, officially and unofficially.

Walking through Suspect on the way to Confirmed, the day's first ambulance arrived and no less than four people were being attended to in the admissions area by a phalanx of anonymous white suits. Conditions were now on the edge of being crowded, the cleaning crews falling behind judging by the number of slop buckets out in the yard.

In Confirmed, our first patients were the Kargbo family and Sally. None of them turned to look up at us, the group sharing three mattresses

pediatric patients in the other buildings, now present to take care of the three Kargbo children with proper pediatric dosing. Alonzo and I coaxed Paracetamol, Valium and metoclopromide into the adults, hoping to lessen their pain, anxiety and nausea. Judging by the amounts of fluids on the floor, we weren't having much luck. It would be a disaster to not have cleaners and sprayers inside to empty the tens of buckets of human waste, spraying down the spills to keep the sewage at a minimum.

Outside on the front deck, the kids recovering, or not yet in the worst throes of the disease, played with toys we had been bringing in or kicking around a soccer ball. Just looking, one could easily think these kids were equal in their wealth of health. I knew better, knowing that some made it through the worst and were going home to regular lives. The others, in the very beginnings, were maybe in the last days of their lives, still able enough to kick a soccer ball. Out of the five children in front of me engaged in horseplay, there was the horrible chance that two were entering the shadows towards the finite. One day, the boy in blue shorts plays games and has friends he looks forward to seeing at school, maybe has a crush on his teacher, or can't sleep as he excitedly waits for morning to check fishing nets with his favorite uncle. Then it stops.

What do they get from us? Back in the States, the vast majority in my profession have careers that provide enough for modest homes, more clothes and groceries than we need, transportation where we spend to status and electronics that are redundant. We have instant mail, voice and internet access on three or four devices, then complain about season ticket prices going up for football games or the price of golf course membership. Pile on the fact that there is a strong cabal of citizens who are quite well off that openly envy the lesser haves, convinced they would have even greater wealth if the lesser haves had less. What sort of person is it who has great fortune that envies the poor man who gets a hand up from the church food pantry? I'd say it's likely the same person that if you asked how much money would be enough for their own wants would reply, "More." Would that person deny these kids having soccer balls on our dime? Probably not. But I know for a fact, because it was told to me to my face by several people, that we were wasting our time and money, nothing would change, etc. There are enough people in this world who do think like that and they are a critical mass, attempting to prove their point by denigrating this type of work, going so far as to use their power and life's achievement to block efforts, spending entire days laboring to stop a child, like the one in front of me in blue shorts, from using "their" wealth. The fact that this boy might only have a week left is all the reason more they see a waste, a bad "investment", as if there is a right of fiduciary return to his very existence. The nuns and priests of my elementary years have such people in their prayers. From us, the boy in the blue shorts gets prayers, spare change and our spare time, the time left over after taking care of ourselves above and beyond our needs.

The five of us headed to doffing, coughing and burning all the way. It was a good round. No corpses. Outside, workers milled about their normal meeting tree, fairly quiet compared to most other days when there would be laughing and teasing going back and forth. George was writing, his attention focused on the clipboard in his lap.

I went down the walk and out the gate to take a bench in the shade of the fence, wanting to decompress a bit before lunch by watching the world drive up and down the road. As I sat resting my wet, sweaty self, two younger fellows in street clothes came down the path, stopping at the guard shack to talk to J Edgar. I noticed he was pointing in my direction at one point in their conversation, likely giving them directions to the entrance. I would normally be curious, but not today. I just wanted some quiet time.

Both men headed towards me, trying to make eye contact. I avoided it as much as possible, focusing on the remaining post of the of the grass hut burned down earlier by the seasonal fires. Both men came into my line of sight and stopped.

The taller one, tan lines around his neck, sporting a fresh crewcut, dressed in a plaid shirt buttoned to the top. His entire outfit looked like he was run over by an REI rack: 200 dollar hiking boots, 150 dollar hiking pants and belt sporting a top of the line multitool. Nice threads. His friend was more casual: big box store jeans, big box store working boots and a blue-black plaid on white shirt from Anystore, America. He wasn't worried about his hair, but it was passable. He assumed a position with his hands behind his back. I assumed they must be with one of the aid groups.

"Hi," the taller one greeted me. "I'm William."

His partner stepped forward, keeping his hands behind his back, bowing slightly as he introduced himself, saying, "I'm James. Nice to meet you."

"Nice to meet you James, William," I replied, not very enthusiastically, wanting my quiet time back.

The taller one, William, took the lead, saying, "The police officer down there told us to come and talk to you. We're hoping you can help us out."

"Well, not help us so much as let us help the afflicted in their time of need," James followed.

I chuckled. "Afflicted? Yeah, you can certainly say they've been afflicted. Almost in an Old Testament sort of way, unfortunately."

"So you're a Christian?" William asked, forcing his smile.

"Raised Catholic," I replied, becoming suspicious. I've met enough people over the years who claim Catholics aren't Christians. In light of Christian history, that's about as remarkably as dumb a thing anyone can say." Then I turned the tables away from giving a straight answer, asking the pair, "What about you two fellows. What's your role here in all this?"

James jumped right in, feet, answering, "We're with a ministry, a Christian aid group that's been in Africa for three generations. Our church back in California was looking for volunteers. We both always wanted to do a mission, bring the Word to the rest of the world. We feel that God has called us and here we are, answering that call."

"Somebody give out your cell phone number?" I quipped. Neither of the pair smiled.

Why anyone would go half around the globe to proselytize about religion baffled me since just about anywhere you go in the world there's religion, sometimes in such abundance they want to share it with us.

Religion is something that can be fashioned to fit your circumstances, made clear in your own mind, free from coercions and pollutions unless the coercions and pollutions had your permission to be part of a paradigm you constructed. Politics eventually demands external expression by your consent into a larger group and seeks to influence the larger community. Make no mistake, much of religion is a sort of an informal politics.

I tried to atone for my joke by feigning interest, saying, "Interesting. You made it to Sierra Leone in one piece. Where are you fellows staying?"

"Freetown. We hired a driver to bring us in for the days and coordinate with a local pastor," William replied. "Our church has a sister church here in Port Loko we support."

"Well, good. You aren't flying blind then," I observed.

James stepped into the conversation, "No, sir, we are not. God has given us a vision," He sounded very much like someone you'd here on AM radio breathing fire and brimstone over the airwaves. "What the pastor told us was you needed help out here. We'd like to help."

"Yes, sir," William concurred. "We understand that, tragically, many are dying from Ebola. As you probably know, Sierra Leone is only about 15% Christian. Now, it isn't hard to do the math, but that would make about 5 out of 6 of your patients not Christian. There isn't anything worse than being on the doorstep of death, facing eternal judgment and not to have been saved. Many of those dying will never know the eternal joy and love of God. We want to fix that."

I was getting a sense of where this was going and it wasn't plausible if my intuition was accurate. "Well, I think you'd have more success by coordinating with your pastor to go out in the community and do what it is you do before they end up here. By the time they get to us, you have a pretty narrow window," I explained, hoping to dissuade them from answering their call here.

Then James verbalized my suspicions, saying, "What we're looking for is to be able to speak with the people inside, the patients, and baptize them into eternal life. We know the risks but we know, too, we can be dressed to be protected. All we'd need is one day a week. Can you help us?"

There it was, right on the ground in front of me, the big egg they just laid. I put my most diplomatic foot forward, saying, "Well, there's no way anyone is going to let you two guys in unless you're medical personnel or trained cleaners or sprayers. The organizations participating in this have huge liabilities trying to keep workers safe. They'll only take on those who have a direct action in patient care and then take on only as many people as they need, not one person more. There's just no way they would consent to the risk of you going in."

"Don't you think their spiritual health is as important as their earthly health?" James asked, hoping to corner me into changing my mind.

"That's the wrong question," I responded, defending my many anonymous patients. "Everyone inside here, every patient, has a religion. It may not be your idea of the perfect religion, but it is theirs. Who am I, or you or you," I said, pointing to all of us, "to make that judgment that their faith, or whatever it is they claim, is inadequate. Everybody inside here is distressed, afraid. What they are enduring is beyond the comfort of anything faith provides. They want to be well and whole again, to go home. Believe me when I say this, every person inside there is praying for a miracle. For many of them that miracle isn't coming. All they have left is hope. Hope is real because it imagines scenarios where they find an answer or someone helps them find the answer. Right now, today, the only hope they have is those of us that go inside give them medicines that offer a fighting chance. It's far from perfect and I'd change a hundred things if I could, but when I see those white suits go through that door, they're taking things in a bag that are a real hope. Belief is for how you live a life. Medicine is so you can just live; they're all at that point: just trying to live."

James quickly responded, raising his voice to accentuate his point, "And we can help take away that fear by giving them the confidence that accepting salvation will give them eternal life."

They weren't going away and it was beginning to annoy me, causing me to snap, "That's presumptuous. It's condescending. What you plan to sell them...."

"Sell them?" William objected.

"Yes, sell them," I countered. "You're offering a product where no one can be held accountable. Whatever failure besets is dismissed as a failure on their part, not a defect in your product. These people are vulnerable and desperate. I honestly can't think of a worse time to try and change someone's mind about something that is so important to them."

"I don't like that word 'sell', "James pleaded. "It sounds like were selling cable subscriptions."

"Let me ask you this straight up," I piped up to both. "Do you think that their being Muslim, animists, whatever, is wrong? Do you think that's something that needs to be fixed?"

William clasped his hands then put them in his rear pockets, thinking, then answering, "They can never know God."

"And you do?" I asked. "As far as many of them are concerned, they think you don't know God, that what you know is all wrong. Think about that: everybody thinks the other guy is wrong. Maybe you're both right. But maybe you're both wrong. Maybe one is right and the other isn't. And the sad part is this: there's no third party to adjudicate which of you of is right and which is wrong, leaving you in a 4000 year old standoff."

"It isn't like those other faiths are representing themselves well to the world," James replied. "They're on a murder spree."

"And the last 2000 years Christians haven't acquitted themselves so well, either," I said. "This isn't the place or time for a battle of the hearts and minds of converts."

James and William were not at all persuaded by my diatribe. Why should they be? They had unshakable certainty, thick walls that repelled all ideas that might plant seeds of doubt, a disciplined inclination to maintain the integrity of their faith in spite of the crushing ignorance that too often was a side effect. They insisted there was no ambiguity in their message, but refused to admit they could not be held accountable thanks, specifically, to ambiguity. A promise of everlasting life is the perfect contract. Dead people hold no one accountable and live people have no proof of eternal life, but that matters nothing since no one is complaining that the goods promised haven't been delivered. The certainty of some people's faith is more important than the faith itself, that what they believe is qualified fact where even the suggestion of verification is apostasy. Many worship the Bible or Quran more than God Himself, precisely because the books are tangible and accessible. God can only be heard when you're abnormally quiet, and even then no one is ever sure of what they heard. For some, orthodox faith is like building a house then never pushing on the walls or double checking the electrical connections to make sure it doesn't collapse on your head in a burning heap. It's much easier to avoid attempts to reconcile the deficiencies.

"So you're saying no to our request?" William asked.

I looked at him, laughing a little, apologizing for the mistake of me as someone who could do such a thing, explaining, "I'm sorry, but I have no control over any sort of request. There are people above me who'd make those calls. I'm more than a little sure they would not approve your request. I can put you in touch with Dr. George but his highest priority is worker safety. I know he'd never allow unnecessary personnel inside. He just can't take that risk or spare the extra bodies to guide you."

"Can you introduce us to him?" William asked, slightly hopeful.

"Sure, I can. But I'm promising nothing," I offered, then continued, hoping to avert wasting Dr. George's time. "Why don't you simply pray for them? Come out here and give this place a blessing? It would be a beautiful gesture. Better yet, what you can do is help the people discharged from here. There are some who are found not infected and sent out with literally nothing—no money, no clothes of their own, no ride home, nothing to eat. It would be great if someone could step up to lend those people a hand."

James waved off my suggestion, saying, "We're not that sort of aid organization. Our mission is people's souls." With that, James, who kept both hands out of sight behind his back throughout our conversation, brought out from behind his back a Bible, well worn in the binding, little colored reference tabs scattered up and down the textblock. He held it out, saying, "This is all anyone needs—The Word of God."

With that, I held my tongue and went to find Ali to ask him if Dr. George came in today. Ali said no but checked his temperature record book to make sure, running his finger down the pages, shaking his head.

I went back outside to a waiting William and James to tell them that Dr. George wasn't in and I had no idea when he would be, explaining that he split his time between Maforki, the Port Loko hospital and several other clinics in the district. By their body language and their eyes, they suspected I was giving them the brush off. I wasn't but I wasn't at all disappointed that Dr. George wasn't in, either. Then I offered a suggestion, saying, "That pastor you're staying with? I think you need to talk to him about the religious dynamics in this country. I'm pretty sure he has quite a few non evangelical friends he sees every day. I'm new here, too, and we all have quite a bit to learn."

"Not about this," James confidently replied, revealing exactly who I thought he was. William was more circumspect, holding his opinion and neither confirming nor denying James.

Both men turned, leaving on foot and heading back towards town, passing by a discharge ceremony out front by the Memory Tree where four survivors were taking turns tying their own ribbons to branches with diminishing free space. William waved at the small crowd but James kept his head down, refusing to acknowledge the gathering since they likely did not fit the profile of the persons his outreach was attempting to bring into the fold. Maybe he was concerned about the well being of the Maforki patients, or maybe he was more interested in his spiritual stature, viewing it as a win-win for both he and his potential converts. Either way, the plotted attempt was a play on a fearful and desperate population likely willing to try anything in their darkest hour. It was a sales pitch where the customer could never make a claim on the warranty, the exact same method used by hucksters who pedal weight loss remedies or cancer "cures", using words of reputation like "doctor" and "researchers" along with concocted testimonials from people who never seem to have a last name. It reminded me of a quote on the wall of my father's car dealership office by some fellow named Ruskin: "There is nothing that cannot be made a little cheaper and sold for a little less. And for the man who considers only price, he is the salesman's lawful prey." Everything is a negotiation. Everything is for sale.

From where I sat outside the fence under the Cuban flag, my attention was taken off the discharge ceremony by the sound of someone speaking, a single voice giving a speech or some sort of rally address. It sounded like George. He continued on, using language that I wasn't familiar with but sounded like Krio. He kept this up for several minutes without interruption, then his voice stopped and the normal chatter of the workers that I was used to hearing returned, absent the usual laughter and verbal horseplay that was perpetual.

J Edgar and two of his subordinate police officers came out from the gate, surprising me since I hadn't seen them go in. I thought he was still down the way in his guard shack. He was looking straight ahead, phone to his ear as he walked by with a determined pace, gesturing to other officers to join him as he walked down the front path of the outer fence. At the guard shack, about six others in navy blue uniforms and black boots surrounded J Edgar, standing in such a way that one could surmise the hierarchy and each person's place within without having to identify their rank by the insignia they wore. Maybe some property had gone missing, the distressed owner believing it was theft, which would be odd in light of the fact that, to my knowledge, nothing had ever been stolen in Maforki.

I went in for lunch, receiving my parcel from the same grumpy lady who had the incredible knack of making me feel guilty for even thinking I deserved a lunch. The usual phalanx of women surrounding her was subdued, talking only as the job required. Many worked 10-hour days putting together meals for the patients. At least a few were required to don gear to deliver the meals. Also, days off were rare to nonexistent, the strain of unending days was taking time away from other life matters that suffered from lack of attention due to the outsized chunks of time consumed by labor. Like the national nurses and the sprayers, most found it easier to live at Maforki rather than waste time walking an hour or more one way every day, using their phones to settle whatever a phone call allowed. Sometimes a family member would come out to speak with a worker to resolve personal issues, knowing the family member would be too inconvenienced to try to take time away.

I ate lunch, wondering if I should bring it to the attention of anyone else what was being proposed by the two missionaries, deciding to keep it to myself, knowing their request would be denied, and that my relaying of the message would only burden those managing the hundred other things that kept us running. Right now, keeping materials and people available and plugged into the right places was an all-consuming job for the various aid organizations trying to co-ordinate efforts. Arranging for a religious mission would mean covering all sorts of ground involving diplomacy, logistics and training, probably even a couple of meetings on what protocols should be written or incorporated into such a request. Keeping my mouth shut would result in a merciful euthanizing of an idea that had all the markings of bad form.

Under the sprayer's shade tree, men were in tight groups, talking and eating lunch, picking at fish buried under mounds of white rice. Some men were filtering in and out of the prayer area for dhuhr, midday prayers, leaving or joining in with those who gathered under the tree. George moved between them, answering questions, shaking his head in disagreement or affirmation, depending on whom he was speaking with at the time, the tone of the conversations sometimes sharp but always with passion and persuasion, George emphasizing various points by shaking a tight fist or slapping his hands.

As I was lazing away the end of lunch hour, Dr. Dahna was outside the supply room digging through a pile of boots, trying them on until she finally found a pair small enough, enabling her to get rid of the pair she had that flopped on her feet. It was as good as time as any to put together the afternoon to-do list and ready supplies we'd need with us.

As I rummaged through the materials in the supply room and reported my takings to the clerk who kept the running inventory, another of the clerks started on my case about a couple of cans of cola I'd taken several days previous for two of the patients. The soda was bought and paid for by the organization, expressly for patients as a treat to help break the monotony and distract from the conditions inside the unit. The older fellow who placed himself in charge of the supply room over the previous weeks, now assumed ownership over the soda. He wanted 10k Leones for the two cans, something I loathed doing since it would be an admission of abdication regards product purchased for patients with organization money. I was polite, but firm, just as I had been over the past days when he demanded payment. The contest was now to see who could wear the other down first.

I went about bagging pharmacy supplies, then headed back to the nurses' station to premix and cobble a medication administration schedule as best I could from memory. The two binders we had been using to try to record what we'd done inside were incomplete, had irrelevant records of discharged or deceased patients, or had none at all on some patients. There simply was no contest between the bedside chart, recorded in immediate time and left near the patient, versus the binders that we tried to fill out from memory. Some of us took notes and tried taping them to the fence to attempt a record from the outside. Others used phones to snap pictures of their taped notes to the fence with varying degrees of success on the resolution. All of us had the problem of finding a decent way to clip the hot zone notes down so they wouldn't blow away. A hot zone whiteboard helped but didn't have enough room for every patient to be charted, leaving yet another hole for our memories to fill, a hole that seemed to be getting deeper and harder to fill with the recent surge of patients. The best way was to recognize what drugs were used and how often, then walk in with an estimate of how much would be needed of this antibiotic or that antimalarial. As long as we were all conscientious about hot zone inventory, paid attention to the bedside chart after each contact, and made sure to fill out the assessments and medication administration records in real time, it worked.

With the morning shift Cubans done with their 6 hour shift, Dr. Dahna and I had no one scheduled with us for the afternoon, freeing us from organizing before hand and working around the labyrinth of time consuming language barriers. Dr. Dahna came back from the national nurses' station, her shiny new boots squeaking up the new concrete walkway poured the day before, to tell me that our assigned national nurse was not making the round with us, saying, "It's just you, me and a sprayer. The nationals are acting all weird, saying they don't know what's going to happen, that we should wait."

I was as puzzled as Dahna, questioning, "What might happen that we have to wait?"

"I think they're just tired, maybe," Dahna surmised. "They're always here, if the smell of their nurses' station means anything."

"I think they need an expanded laundry facility," I remarked. "But first they need a laundry facility to expand. I've seen workers take showers in their work clothes to wash them, then hang' em on the fire pit fence to sun dry. You'd never guess it from how good they always look."

Dahna gave me a distracted nod of agreement, her focus on our list, adding notes and ideas. We donned not in the usual chaos; it was observably less so without the nationals, but no one really gave it a second thought as all the sprayers were bi and tri lingual and, in a pinch, were adequate translators and interpreters.

Outside, George was relentlessly moving between people. Out of place and not at their normal post, though, was J Edgar and another officer, inside the gate at the check in station, passively standing and watching.

Racin was our sprayer. Rather than his normal jocularity of with anyone within 100 yards of him, he was keeping to himself, all business about the hot zone plan we'd thrown together. I poked at him, "Racin, why so glum?"

Racin shook his head, walked over to me and opened his mouth, putting his index finger on one of his molars, then garbled, "Toothache. Can you give me some Cipro for it? Please, I need it."

The cavity was obvious. I waved over Dr. Dahna to look at Racin. She poked at the side of his face, causing him to wince, then concurred, saying, "I'll set up some Cipro for you and some Paracetamol when we finish."

Racin thanked her and finished donning but stopped us as we started to step towards the hot zone walkway, saying, "We need to hurry. There might be no sprayers coming out."

"What do you mean?" I asked.

"We sprayers are going on strike. George is setting it up now. I think it will start in about an hour," Racin stated matter of factly.

"Strike? Seriously?" Dahna asked back, continuing, "we better have someone to clean us up or we're going to be stuck."

"No worry. No one will be left behind," Racin assured us. "We just want to get the attention of Dr. George and get him to talk to us."

Dahna and I exchanged a look, anxious to get going. The inconsistent schedules, job duties and paydays for the nationals were an open secret, with everyone assuming it was being handled. George, and others, felt it wasn't being handled, and the three day lock down period only served to lengthen the time for reaching a resolution.

We made rounds with Racin in tow, disinfecting us after each contact and helping us with the non English speaking patients. No one was concerned about the bubbling rumors of a walkout by national staff since we were powerless to stop it, even if we wished. The contingency plan was 'wait and see what happens', as good as any since only at the time something happens is the true nature of an event understood. Prior plans to deal with massive disruptions are usually no more than educated guesses, the only upside being there is a chain of command assigned to confront a disaster. The first response for those involved is to know what they are responding to and establishing reliable means of verifying information for decision-making, a monumental task when the usual means of relating become disrupted. Then again, we were probably burying our heads in the sand with the 'wait and see' approach, hoping the workers would back off.

Inside, we were unaware of the commotion, focused on work. Only when we finished did we hear the shouting and chants in the general yard. George's voice rose above all else. From behind the chain link fence of the doffing area, standing in my bucket of bleach for the required minute, I could see George raise his arm, holding up all 5 fingers then one by one folding them into his palm to form a fist he would pump into the air as others shouted.

It was apparent Racin was distracted as he sprayed us down, hitting my visor with bleach. He was trying to keep one eye on what was happening outside and one eye on his job, all the while trying to get the rest of the decontamination team to pay attention to us, to get us out without breaching protocol. At the exit, several expatriate staff waited for us, monitoring the doffing process but quietly watching the yard with concern. When Racin was in the final stages of his own doffing, a blue vested NGO worker asked us to immediately head back to the nurses' station. Management met us and explained that sprayers and cleaners were walking out, striking, and that we needed to form into small groups and keep track of one another until the drivers, summoned on a moment's notice, arrived to get us back to our respective compounds.

Looking around the nurses' station, I could see that those usually assigned to support duties over in the admissions' building were with us, a sign that management was viewing this as a serious situation. The usual work chatter was replaced with questions about was happening, how long the whole ordeal might last and how this would affect patient care.

If we thought it was loud when the workers were engaged in their protests, it was nothing compared to what happened next when soldiers clad in blue camouflage, armed with AK-47's, opened up the main gate and marched in, led by J Edgar and his police officers. Battle lines formed. A milling crowd of workers faced the soldiers in formation, hurling insults at those protecting the menace responsible for skipped paydays and broken schedules. J Edgar, bullhorn in hand, looked over the crowd, then retreated to consult with what appeared to be a commanding officer.

J Edgar turned from the soldiers and waded back into the crowd, looking to see who he could speak to, going person to person until he finally settled at George. George, his green eyes intense as his body was rigid, emphatically shook his head in the negative at J Edgar's questions or demands, leaving J Edgar and his own contingent looking more worried than the moments before. Judging by the tightly wound body language of the workers, George, police, J Edgar and the soldiers, the situation was ripe for ignition, one side feeling it could not back away without losing the legitimacy of its grievances and the other bound to keep order.

J Edgar backed out of the crowd as they jeered him, then raised his voice, forgoing the bullhorn, shouting, "This is an illegal gathering. It is in violation of the laws of the 3 day lockdown. You must go back to work immediately!"

Whether J Edgar expected this to work or not, I couldn't tell, but the order did nothing but inflame the workers who took several steps towards the line the soldiers formed, causing the soldiers to anxiously look at their commanding officer for direction and pull their weapons in a little tighter. The commanding officer was motionless, keeping his eyes directly on the people in front of him, exercising restraint moment to moment, likely knowing that violence at an Ebola treatment unit would be a disaster.

The workers' shouts crescendoed, adding further to the tension and confusion. Some workers were now bluffing the soldiers with fast motions, mimicking a charge, while the calmer ones grabbed the backs of the shirts of their more aggressive colleagues to rein them in. George stood at the front, in the middle, as loud as anyone, taunting the enforcement teams, then turning to rally his fellow sprayers and cleaners to keep up the din.

J Edgar's eyes moved back and forth across the crowd and settled on George. J Edgar stepped back to take an audience with the commanding officer. No sooner had the two finished their conversation then J Edgar moved with decisive steps directly towards George, grabbed him by both arms, turned him and held George's wrists and hands together so one of his officer's could thread and tighten a tie strap, arresting him. George went to the ground, struggling against the hands of the officers. The workers went silent for a second or two, then began screaming insults at the top of their lungs. Some moved close in, hoping to scare off the police to reclaim George, but J Edgar picked George off the ground and kept him facing the crowd, using George as a shield.

The commanding officer, who had been verbally restrained, broke his silence and shouted over the crowd for them to disperse. Fully expecting a lack of compliance, he immediately followed his first order with a second for his soldiers to shoulder arms. The dozen of them hesitated, and then complied, looks of dread at what they might be ordered to do in the next seconds.

Outside the gate, someone spotted our vehicles and drivers. J Edgar ordered us to skirt the crowd and take our rides. Several policemen escorted us off to the right to create a shield from the showdown happening in front of us, seeing to it that we all loaded. From the back of the minivan, we could hear the shouting continue. Musa and Ibrahim translated the Krio for us, explaining that the workers were demanding an immediate release of George, who was now behind locked doors in a police van that pulled out and was heading to Port Loko prison. Having driven by the prison more than a few times, it appeared to be a pretty awful place with dirty gray stone walls, rusty concertina wire and black steel doors, the sort of place where if you go in you likely did not come out the same person--or maybe even a live person. I liked George. And I was worried about George.

After Ibrahim drove us down the road to the Total gas station, the closest thing to a convenience store like one back in the States, everyone released a collective sigh, realizing that our anxiety was on the high side as it eased back the further down the road we drove. Inside the station, someone from the group decided that the organization owed us a couple of drinks, peeling off a roll of Leones after setting an armload of cold beers on the counter. Back in the van, the pop of metal tabs was near simultaneous as everyone took a couple of slugs off their drinks.

The trip back into town was early for the day, meaning we had about two hours of extra free time. As we crossed the bridge, I watched the children swimming at the bottom of the river rapids, their mothers beating away on laundry. Up the road, we passed the Imam's house, reminding us that we had gotten a blessing that morning and no one really knew what it was.

Inside the compound, we shared some snacks from our personal stashes while Adam cruised the net, trying to find verses in an online Quran as the internet turned into the intermittent net during the lockdown. After a good half hour, Adam found the verses, and read:

" 'It was then that God made the infant Jesus speak from the cradle and he spoke of his prophecy for the first time. Jesus said: "I am indeed a servant of Allah: He hath given me revelation and made me a prophet; And He hath made me blessed wheresoever I be, and hath enjoined on me Prayer and Charity as long as I live; He hath made me kind to my mother, and not overbearing or miserable; So peace is on me the day I was born, the day that I die, and the day that I shall be raised up to life again!' Verses 19:30-33 in the Quran's Mary chapter."

After unraveling what was read, the juxtaposition of the blessing in contrast to the events of the day was the one amusing thing that had happened. Merry Christmas had become Exciting Christmas, but no one was dead, so it was now a thankful Christmas. For poor George, we were all certain that his incarceration was hardly the plan he had for holiday. The hope was that everything would be resolved quickly enough and George would be home by sunset. In the meantime, the rest of work would continue, oblivious to the hiccup.

■■

Changing Gears

The countrywide Christmas lockdown achieved....fill in the blank. Opinions varied from all angles. My own personal view is that it was not the normal everyday business of commerce in the marketplace that was spreading the disease, but the normal proximity of family and village where personal contact is always part of the day. There is no difficulty avoiding direct contact in commerce because it is objects that are the focus of transactions. With burials, children, an ill friend or family member, human contact is expected and considered healthy, be it to mourn, cure or comfort. The opposite argument is that sick people travel, too, and by limiting travel, you limit spread.

Either way, we were at an apex, admissions running in the teens and twenties everyday while outlying Critical Care Clinics, CCC's, were picking up their fair share as well. Still, judging by the numbers in the District Emergency Response Center and National Emergency Response Center reports, many Ebola victims were being identified as such only after their death, not picked up in the still evolving contact tracing efforts. The increasing numbers stretched staff, but overall there had been a steady increase in responders, enough that a regular evening and night shift were able to be staffed at Maforki, filling a gaping hole in continuity of care that previously left patients alone for up to 12 hours daily, even with national nursing staff on grounds 24/7.

I was on the evening shift the day after Christmas along with one other expatriate nurse, joining the national nursing staff and other support staff. Any worries about having enough sprayers and cleaners had been put to rest with a Christmas night negotiation session that addressed striking workers' concerns. One demand was George was to be released the following morning, in good condition. If there was no George, there would be no workers. The next morning there was no George, only a promise he would be freed, exposing another frayed end of a fuse ignition point needing prompt address, creating uncertainty where none should've existed.

The kinks in the added shifts became apparent before the start, namely that I was out of the lunch loop. With lockdown still in effect, simply going to the market circle for a quick bite was a nonstarter with all servers closed. Going hungry during the day was no big deal since there would be supper at work, but the lack of daytime electricity in the rooms at the Ghetto meant the loss of the fan and the presence of stale air. Fortunately, humidity was low and the temperature was maybe mid-80's, giving me time to finish up my overdue library books 8000 miles from their assigned shelves.

With second shift, you're always going to work the entire day, losing the relaxation that comes from accomplishing a job that allows a person to wind down, to think or forget, depending on what transpired. Second shift gives you plenty of waking hours to feed anxiety.

I arrived at Maforki with my fellow second shift nurse, picked up at the Dutch camp, where I got a rundown on an elaborate six-course meal served Christmas day at their compound. The contrast was striking to our Christmas day spread at the Ghetto but the company my group comprised was interesting and respectful, a friendly informality. If you look forward to seeing someone at the end of the day, there is no more sure sign you're in the right place. If I were in the Dutch camp, there would be the natural segregation of groups by nationality and the constant forced formality and uncertainty over etiquettes. Would I have to quietly learn the finer points of European football, or would it be OK to ask what assuredly would be obvious to an Englishman or Belgian? Could I wear my scrubs to breakfast, or would they judge me fit only for a leper colony? Is there an unwritten curfew, a disdain of discussing work on off hours? Small enough matters, but in the short term, a few stumbles over such trivial items can add up to a person being viewed as a prima donna or a lumbering social dimwit. No, the old shoe fit. Maybe not stylish, but familiar.

I learned immediately that my fellow nurse was unable to join me inside the hot zone, disabled with what looked like a bad hip and an accompanying limp. Neither of us knew what to expect, nor was I worried about what to expect. Our primary duty would be to make rounds, see to it that medication schedules were followed and developing symptoms given relief as patients needed. You could never go wrong hanging another IV and cleaning someone up. The only complication was that we were a team of two nurses and a sprayer, trying to care for sixty some odd patients between admissions.

Second shift was not spared admissions, which continued to run high. Mary and I made the fatal assumption that the majority of the admissions would be handled on day shift. That assumption evaporated on arrival to the admissions' building. Gwyn and her cohorts were juggling phone calls for eventual arriving ambulances, some estimating their time out as much as four to six hours, deep into second shift. The pair of us had no clue how to perform an admission prior to walking them into the ETU, necessitating a crash course of where to find the paper work, how to fill out forms, enter the necessary computer information for lab requests, fill out patient wrist bands, conduct an admissions assessment for placement or whom to call regards certain unexpected situations. At least now, I knew what to dread all day before second shift, learning that second shift was merely a continuation of first shift minus many, many hands by which to divide the work. Someone, somewhere, was going to have to get the short end of the stick.

Triage, by design, is the exclusion of many for the priority of one, an idea I can rationally accept and defend but, in practice, it is unnerving to inform a patient or worse yet, ignore them completely, that their emergency is not mine. The Good Samaritan stopped to help the injured man on the roadside and it was the injured man's distress that became the Good Samaritan's priority. His easy out was there was only one person needing help. It takes practice to learn to ignore a stranger in need, a decision millions of us make almost daily in large cities, where we learn to ignore the begging homeless because of the impossibility of the one of ourselves saving the all of them.

Gwyn ran us through the entire process. Thankfully, it was all well laid out, the kinks worked out by her and her staff through trial and error and some thoughtful foresight. Mary's not being able to go in with me became a blessing in disguise, giving us each the freedom to focus and master our respective tasks; the division of labor gave me the inside and she the outside. Additionally, several national nurses and sprayers with us for the evening knew their way around well enough to flesh out the body of work.

No sooner than we finished covering process points, it was time to suit up and head inside, an ambulance at the gate, anxious to drop their human delivery and get back on the road to home. I donned entirely in the admissions' building with Josephine's help to make sure I was zipped and sealed. It hadn't been more than 5 minutes and the ambulance driver was shouting unintelligibly to no one in particular, but it was clear he felt the stop was already 6 minutes overdue. A sprayer accompanied me, anonymous in his gear and no name on the apron, forcing me to give him a name so I could get his attention as needed.

The naming process I joked with was embraced with enthusiasm by the nationals, such that I began to think they purposely avoided writing names on their aprons so they could be named, a highlight of their day. I explained to the sprayer he was unknowable under all his gear, that he was dressed in a Halloween costume. Naturally, the cartoon character of Casper the Friendly Ghost came to mind. Casper was perplexed at first, but a little more explaining on my part brought him out of his shell of doubt and he embraced the name, fully satisfied it was something genuinely American. I tried to explain Aaron Rodgers to him but it was clear the Green Bay Packers were as foreign to him as Sierra Leone's top soccer personality was to me. In the meantime, our naming ceremony was aggravating the driver, enough so he exited the ambulance. He was greeted with an onslaught of derision and scolding to get back in his cab, lest he carelessly expose himself.

Casper and I approached the back of the ambulance and I sat back to let him do his thing-- spray down the rear doors. I opened the doors and stepped back to allow Casper room to spray the floor and the inside of the doors. He sprayed my hands and boots and only then was I finally allowed close to the rear of the vehicle and peek inside at the arrival. Sitting on the bench sat a twenty something year old man looking perfectly bored, not caring one way or the other he had arrived and that his trip was finished. Casper, speaking Krio, summoned the man to the back of the ambulance into the sunlight, allowing me to make my first visual assessment. His eyes were red but he was able to walk and speak with no difficulties, so having him step off and down to take a chair under the shade of the admissions' tarp was easy enough.

Over the fence, a national nurse began her assessment questions in Krio, leaving me out of the loop, but not for long, since she was eventually able to hold up the assessment form for me to take direction. While she was asking questions, I was recording a temperature, taking a radial pulse and looking for other signs and symptoms of infection around the mouth, eyes and nose. Once we both finished our piece of the assessment, she again held up the completed form for me to read. It was clear he had been in close contact with at least one relative who had recently died of Ebola infection, having participated in the washing of the body prior to burial.

Josephine was finished writing out the wrist band so I asked her to ask him if anyone ever related it was dangerous to wash the corpse of an Ebola victim. They exchanged words of Krio that went on longer than a one or two questions, then Josephine relayed his answers to me, saying, "They had three people come to the village to help with the Ebola and they were asked to listen. They were talked to for a long time but no one would answer questions about malaria medicines or help with sleeping nets. Their medicine women told them they would be protected if their belief in God was strong and they respected the dead. Some in the village felt the workers were making fun of the beliefs, or trying to get them to believe like whites so they could sell things or get cheap workers. He decided to believe the people that stayed, not the ones who came, and then left."

You can't argue with that. A total stranger arrives, offers advice but no help. Antimalaria medicines are cheap and hugely appreciated, a guarantee of good intentions. The aid workers came with nothing, not even a book whose pages they could use to start a fire, not an uncommon use of some of the literature left by missionaries to people English illiterate. Yet, the overall messages on Ebola safety were gradually taking hold, the proof being that certain families and villages were expelling or isolating the sick but going overboard in extending the expulsions to survivors.

I finished wrist banding our new patient, took his bucket of admission materials and led him into a Suspect ward. Inside, Casper found an empty bed for the man and helped explain the importance of drinking water, and that people would come to draw blood to test for Ebola and malaria. His anxiety was obvious in how he scanned the rest of the room. I fished out 10mg of diazepam and some acetaminophen.

Casper and I stepped outside to head to doffing but ended being waved back over to the admissions area. Gwyn was finishing up her day and wanted to bring me up to speed on what to expect, ticking off her notes about incoming ambulances that took several minutes to finish.

"That's a total of how many?" I asked.

"5 ambulances with at least 5 patients," Gwyn casually informed.

"When do they get here?" I asked, worried about how I would fit a normal round in between admissions.

"One is outside now with one patient. The others will likely be arriving in the next two to 6 hours. You'll have to use national nurses to help you," Gwyn advised, hoping to assuage my concerns.

"Nationals are off at 8 o'clock. What happens after that?" I wondered outloud.

Gwyn was sympathetic, saying, "I know. Maybe you can get one of them to help you. This is the first day we're taking admissions around the clock and this is our first day of evening and night shift. We'll have more people, eventually."

I knew about the shifts. What I didn't know for certain was if the national nursing staff had their duty hours expanded, though, in their defense, there weren't enough of them to perform such an expanded modification of hours. I wasn't disappointed either way, but it was a revelation that we would be taking all comers around the clock. In our weekly update meeting, I must have missed this piece of information, but doubted it since I was the first evening shift, breaking new ground and wanting to get it right. The expectation was that I would assist with late afternoon admissions and do a patient round later in the evening. In hindsight, my skepticism had gone AWOL, not grasping the amount of time it would take for a single admission, much less several, or where the patient may be too disabled, requiring raw muscle and extra diligence to treat their presenting symptoms. It is one thing to deal with a walking, talking patient who is alert and oriented, quite another to help someone who is too weak to walk, confused and needs to be hit with every treatment available to give them a fighting chance.

I waved Gwyn off, trying to reassure her and myself as well, saying, "Somehow we'll figure this out. There's always going to be bumps and dips. The worst that happens is we do admissions all night. It'd be nice to make a round; maybe that's a luxury we can fix tomorrow. At least those coming in are going to get started on treatments instead of waiting until tomorrow."

Gwyn agreed. "Focus on the admissions. Sometimes they call and tell us they're coming, then don't until the next day. Don't be surprised if half of them don't show."

Laughing through my sweat, I shouted back, "Won't hurt my feelings at all if they wait until tomorrow. Have a good evening."

Gwyn left Casper, Josephine and me at the fence. Mary was inside, tearing up cloth for rags, putting together admission buckets, recording our newest patient's information onto whiteboard tags and entering lab orders into the phlebotomists' register. This was as good as a division of labor as any, saving all of us the stress of donning and doffing and running around to do bookwork and patient care. Casper and I were the odd men in for the night, Mary and a national nurse in charge of the charting.

I was thinking of heading out when Josephine yelled across the fence. "Another ambulance." She then retreated inside the admissions building and out came a half-suited national, waiting until the ambulance docked before finishing donning.

Casper and I waited on the dock as the large gates opened and the Red Cross/Red Crescent ambulance backed in, its blue light flashing for no good reason. The driver shouted back and forth with several of the nationals opposite of our fence, seeming annoyed. Apparently, when ambulance drivers are hired, being surly is considered a job requirement. Casper sprayed the rear doors, then me, before I opened the doors. The amount of bleach the ambulances were being sprayed with was taking its toll on the hardware, corroding the hinges and locks, oxidizing them stiff.

Inside was a mother with child of about 4 years of age. The kid was sitting upright on the gurney but mom was flaccid, stirring only slightly from the noise of me opening the door. I reached for the child but the little girl pulled back from me, afraid. Casper was doing his best to calm the girl and it was working, leaving her whimpering rather than bellowing out a full-throated scream. Eventually, Casper's soothing prodding worked and the child allowed me to take her under the arms to lift her out and into one of the waiting white plastic chairs where our national nurse was able to continue reassuring the child.

"Casper," I said, "I know it's not what you normally do but I'm going to need your help maybe."

His enthusiastic response lightened my worry. "No problem. Just tell me what you need."

I hopped up inside to take a closer look at mom. Her tight cornrows were unraveling and her dress lafa was soaked. I tapped her cheek lightly until she turned her head to look at me. She whispered something unintelligible then averted her gaze to take in the surroundings, lifting her head with difficulty to look out the back of the ambulance. She caught sight of her child, then let her head fall back onto the gurney mattress. I hopped back down and grabbed the gurney bar to lift and unlock it from the floor. The weeks of bleaching had destroyed the locks and it took several good tugs to break it free before the gurney rolled forward with my pull, then dropped and locked its wheels. Now the driver started shouting again.

Casper stepped around me and began shouting back, the two of them making a not so joyful noise, leaving me relieved I couldn't understand, making my arguing needless. With my socks soaked in my boots with my own sweat, I could feel them squishing, the heat of the gear was starting to catch up, causing me to remind myself that as a distance runner I challenged myself routinely with late afternoon August workouts, often when heat and humidity were in the 90's. If I did that for fun, I reminded myself, I could easily do this for work.

Casper stepped in front of me. "He says you can't keep the gurney."

I laughed, telling Casper, "I know that. Just for fun, tell him we sell them to the brothels."

Before I could stop Casper, he started shouting back in Temne exactly what I asked him to do. The driver was caught off guard, if his sudden pause was any indication, then he turned to me shouting and pointing at his gurney. I waved him down and Casper yelled at him to not step any further away from the ambulance lest he contaminate himself. Casper reassured the driver he would get his gurney back, but he needed to return to his driver's seat after Casper sprayed the man's hands and boots, which was done, and the driver complied.

I dragged the gurney and mom over close to where the child was sitting and lowered the gurney so child and mother could eye one another. The background whimpering from the child stopped. The national nurse, on the opposite of the fence in full gear, reached out with a scanning thermometer to the child's forehead and recorded a temperature of normal. She proceeded down the triage checklist, eliciting answers from a reluctant child with her maternal touch and verifying them against mom's recollections that required us to be quiet as possible to hear her whispered answers. Mom had a fever, her forearm skin tented with my soft pinch, her lips were dry and cracked, eyes bloodshot and lafa soaked in diarrhea. She was definitely infected and had other family members who were recently stricken with Ebola. No other signs or symptoms were present for the child. I wanted to swear. So I did.

I yelled into the admissions building for Mary to come out, which she did, ready with two admission buckets. Frustrated, I pointed to the child, saying, "This kid just came in with her mom. She has no temp and no other signs or symptoms I can see. Mom's a wreck, so we'll have to start an IV and run her on fluids and antibiotics. But this little girl, she doesn't fit the admission criteria; she's well. Nothing wrong at all—for now."

Mary set down the buckets. "We can't put her in," Mary half scolded me, warning me off even considering it an option, which I didn't.

"How do we handle this?" I asked, looking at the national nurse and Mary. "Maybe Josephine knows something. Josephine!"

Josephine came out, her evening jacket on, ready to leave since her day was over. She tossed aside her supper and joined Mary and the national at the fence.

"Josephine," I half pleaded, "please tell us you know what happens when a sick mom and a well child come in together. Is there a place we call?"

Josephine slowly shook her head, not knowing, then offered what Mary and I should have known immediately. "I would call Musa. He's the social worker. Sometimes he works with the orphanages in Port Loko."

Mary took charge. "I'll get the phone and get Musa." She headed into the building to start putting out our surprise brush fire.

The national nurse called me closer to the fence and offered her plan. "The little one will need to be washed and disinfected and put into new clothes. I will bring all this to you and you do everything right in that chair where she sits. You clean up, then do the cleaning and changing." With that, she disappeared back towards the admission building where Josephine assembled a third bucket with the 0.05% bleach solution, soap, water, drying rags and a fresh blue dress.

Mom watched us, either understanding what was happening or too sick to object. Casper sprayed me down and I rubbed up my arms, the chlorine gas in the bleach tickling my throat and stinging in my eyes. I held out my hands after a minute of soaking so the national nurse could rinse my hands so I wouldn't be touching the child's skin with the harsh cleansers sprayed on me. Taking the bucket of water over the fence, Casper and I tried to coax the little girl to stand in it but she was having none of that, wailing out her objection. We let her go back to the chair. Our next maneuver was to remove her dress, then use a rag Josephine had soaked in mild bleach. I took the rag and at the touch of the rag to the four year olds skin, she flinched, flinching so hard that she began to tip the chair, causing Casper and I both to overreact in trying to stop child and chair from hitting the gravel. Too much, too late. The child fell over the chair arm and landed on her left shoulder, my hand between her head and the gravel. She let out a blood-curdling scream that tightened my entire spine, but the fear that I just failed to protect her was far worse. Mom, relatively inert up to this point, sat up and yelled, reaching out to grab me. Again, my first thought was, 'Don't let her breach you!', so I slapped her hand away and took a step out of her reach. Mary came back outside, on the phone, yelling into it, simultaneously assessing our unfolding mini disaster and settling our situation via Musa.

Casper up righted the chair and I lifted the child into it, blocking out the cacophony of voices admonishing or advising. Either way, it must have worked because Casper and I both had rags of mild disinfectant on her body as she cried, the noise only stopping as she paused to reinflate her lungs for another set of sobbing wails. No scratches or scrapes meant no further complication to an already complicated situation. We followed up the disinfecting wash with soap and water, head to toe, rinsing her down by soaking fresh rags and letting them drip over her head, then wiping her down some more. Mom had fallen back on to her gurney, lucid enough to turn her head into the mattress of the gurney to avoid watching her child squirm under our rags. We finished, dried her and dropped the blue dress over her head. While we had managed not to drown her by way of washing, she was drowning in the blue dress Josephine had selected. But it would do and there was no time to quibble over fittings. Someone had dropped a pair of child-sized sandals over the fence and we slipped her into them.

Casper quickly sprayed my hands, arms and front and let it soak for the required one minute. The national nurse and Josephine brought over more fresh water and rinsed down my hands and arms. Mary, several yards back near the admissions building, was still on the phone, the time that passed indicating there was some confusion over exactly what to do with the child.

We had a clean child who was not ill and did not fit the admission criteria. Putting her inside with her sick mother was not an option. As painful as the separation was going to be, there was no choice except the compassionate one—do not expose the child to any further risk and pray like hell mom makes it so that this isn't this little girl's last memory of Mom, a disabled woman grieving as she sees the last of her child.

The heat was taking its toll on the three of us in gear. You could see it by how deliberate each of us moved, absent the automatic fluidity of motion when a person feels well and strong. The crying child tried to get off the chair and get to Mom, but I caught her under the arms as she was backing on down. I then lifted her in one smooth motion over the fence and into the arms of the other national nurse who in turn handed her to Josephine, who had her game face on, emotionless, and she quickly marched away into the admissions building. Outside, we could hear yelling and screaming, the utter distress of the child rattling the all of us, though no one was letting the person next to them know.

I asked to read the national nurse's notes she managed to get from the mother one more time before taking Mom inside. She had previous contact with other Ebola victims, temperature was 103, eyes blood shot, diarrhea, obviously dehydrated, fatigued and nauseous. The ambulance driver was yelling again, likely wanting to get going home before sunset, which was approaching. Casper attempted to persuade the driver to let us use the gurney to transport the woman into a Suspect ward but the driver was going to have none of that, even though Casper could spray the entire contraption and return it cleaner than it had arrived. Looking about the admission dock, all we had was one crappy rusted out wheel chair and a jury-rigged litter where someone nailed a body bag to two pieces of log.

I examined the litter for sharp ends and snags from the nails used to pin it to the wood. Overall, they were minor and not near the grab points. I talked to mom, apologizing about the child and asked Casper to please tell her that the child looks healthy and will be in a safe place waiting for her when she gets better. Casper squatted next to me, putting his face close to the mother so he would not have to yell, then relayed what I had asked him to say. She nodded her head, knowing she was in no position to object. After that, I straightened her out and rolled her up on to her side while Casper tucked a blanket full length beneath her. We rolled her to the opposite side and pulled the blanket through to use as a lift. On the ground next to the gurney, the slap dash body bag stretcher was in the ready position and we lifted the mother down onto it.

The day's light was dimming but was enough to start an IV. The mother's dehydrated status made her veins smaller and harder to locate, but there was enough good spots to take a poke with the 20 gauge someone tossed in for us. I took her left hand and found the spot, having to take only one go at it. Mary tossed two liters of IV fluid over the fence, landing them on the foot of the stretcher between mom's legs for us to hang when we got her onto a bed.

Casper sat himself on the chair, taking a small rest. His spray pack, weighing about 25 pounds, was slipping off one shoulder by intention, giving his back a quick rest. Before I could ask if he was ready to go, he slipped the sprayer back on and grabbed the head of the stretcher with me following his lead. Fortunately, the woman probably weighed no more than 100 pounds, making the 150 foot walk to S-4, Wet, doable without stopping. Up the concrete ramp and down the walkway we maneuvered until we finally made it to 4. The fluorescent lighting was harsh and not conducive to good sleep, but it allowed us to string the IV line and start the first bag of fluids. With some coaxing, the mother took the offered metoclopromide, Cipro and Paracetamol. I followed that with a dose of oral Valium, hoping to give her some rest, maybe distract her from the separation scenario she had just been through with her child. I titrated the IV drip to run as quickly as possible, hoping to be able to be back within the next hour and a half to start a second bag. After filling out her bedside chart and taking another spray down from Casper, the cool bleach water giving me some respite, I took his spray pack and did the same for him. The both of us were now having the same issue with breathing, our N-95 masks soaked with our own spit and sweat so much that it gurgled with each inhalation and exhalation. But we were going to head out, get a drink, cool off and dry up, so it didn't matter. The end was in sight.

We walked out of the unit, me carrying the litter to return to our admissions dock first before leaving. As I got closer to the gate, I could hear Musa and the others inside, causing a wave of relief to wash over me knowing that his Sierra Leonean roots, and everything that entails, would find a solution for placing the four year old. As I dropped off the litter next to the fence and turned to head out with Casper, I caught a glimmer of flashing blue light, surmising that the ambulance we had just emptied was now out and on its way. As I turned to head to doffing, Josephine called out, yelling, "There is another ambulance coming in!"

I stopped and turned, shouting back, "Are you sure?"

She looked at me, then chastised my doubt, saying, "Why would I say that if it wasn't true?"

"Because you're Josephine and you hate me," I half joked.

Casper, buried beneath his layers of plastic, rubber and Tyvek, slumped a little. Whatever enthusiasm he had, it was fading fast. It wasn't like mine was any better. I wanted a drink of water and to take a mental break, to gather my wits; I could only assume that Casper wanted to do the exact same thing. He was going beyond his job description to help me the way he was since handling patients was not in his job description, that being to simply follow and disinfect as much and as often as possible. I was grateful he wasn't objecting and took advantage of his generosity.

Musa was now at the fence, waving me in. He was in his street clothes, meaning he came from in town where he probably was called away from supper, the thought reminding me that Casper and I probably missed our own suppers. Heat suppresses appetite, so for the time being it was a non issue. Musa was munching on a licorice stick, head down looking at his phone. When I got close enough, he looked up and started filling me in, saying, "We're placing the child at the Catholic orphanage, so you might want to tell that to the mother."

"Oh, good," I uttered, tired.

"You don't sound too happy, man," Musa picked up from my answer.

"Oh, no, that's good you were able to find a place. This wasn't the place for the kid here. Thanks for being able to pull it off because, for awhile, we were all pretty concerned about what to do." I continued, explaining, "I probably just sound a little winded. We've been in awhile. What time is it?"

Musa looked at his phone, then held it up for me to see the time. "That says 7:30. How long you been inside?" Musa asked.

I looked at Casper, nudging him with my elbow for his answer, to which he shrugged, saying, "We went in about 4:30."

Mary joined Musa at the fence, interrupting to say, "There are two ambulances outside. Each one has one patient apiece."

Casper cussed, and not just a little, but I let it roll over me, thinking we could make this fast if the two of them could walk and talk.

"Mary," I half pleaded, "could you have the first ambulance come in now. We'll take the patient and just seat them, get the ambulance out and have the second one come in right away. That way, they get going rather than waiting for us to run through the admission process for the first patient. If you can put together the admission buckets and wrist bands, Josephine and the other national nurse can ask all the questions.

I'll get them started on their meds and IV's."

Everyone agreed and Mary left to arrange it all. We thanked Musa again and he walked off to take care of the child. Casper and I sat ourselves in the plastic chairs, sharing our common complaints of being sweat soaked and greasy, but trying to convince each other that it was seasonably cooler than normal so we were lucky.

Soon enough, both ambulances dropped the patients and everyone pitched in to get all the information. Both were alert and oriented and spoke excellent English, eliminating the time consuming process of reiterating the same question several different ways to ascertain we had the correct information. A flurry of action under flashlights got both young men started on IV's and given their initial doses of medications. Mary and Josephine were able to talk across the fence to get all the health assessment questions answered and recorded, then instructed the men about the bucket contents and when they would be having their blood tested. The entire process felt like it went fast, but the argument against that was now that it was pitch dark out, the only light was from the solar powered LED yard lights', meaning it was getting late.

Casper resumed his normal job duties and followed, focusing on his disinfecting duties as I walked the two young men into a Suspect Dry unit, doing my best to explain when we'd know more about their status and why it was important to drink as much water as possible. For now, neither man needed IV fluids nor any extra help in taking care of their own hygiene needs, freeing Casper and me up to finally leave.

We walked over to Confirmed to head out, but the noise from a radio was at high volume, something that needed to be turned down for everyone's comfort. Inside Confirmed Three, off to the left of the door, was a young man half on and half off his mattress, wallowing in his own waste, his eyes not fixating. I knelt beside him then spoke loudly, hoping I could snap him to attention, but the best I was able to elicit was a brief look before he began scanning again, pretty much oblivious to me. He hiccupped occasionally, his respirations somewhat elevated at about 24 or 28 a minute, his IV pulled out, leaving him oozing blood from his hand where the IV once was, red-black smear everywhere. Was it worth trying to restart it? No. It was very likely he had some type of meningitis beyond treatment and the hiccups were the final sign. I found his chart two beds down and saw that he tested positive for both malaria and Ebola and was getting hammered with IV antibiotics and Artesimin, an antimalaria, over the last four days.

Casper knelt beside me and together we heaved the man back onto his mattress, then rolled him up onto his side so that should he throw up, he wouldn't aspirate, more a precaution not to prevent his death, which was imminent, but to prevent a panicky death by asphyxiation. It took three pulls for the two of us to get him back, the both of us melting in our gear. After cleaning him, we gave him a pillow from some clean rags and covered him with a dry lafa plus a clean heavy blanket that resembled a moving quilt, a rough wool cotton blend that was not the most comfortable item to sleep with to thwart the cool nights, yet worked well in tandem with a lafa sheet. There was a syringe of Valium left over on the med table from an afternoon round, neatly labeled with dose and time, giving me enough confidence the medication hadn't lost any of its efficacy. A quick jab into the thigh rested on the hope that sleep would follow after we left him with for the night.

Josephine Kargbo was sitting upright on her mattress, watching us from across the room. Two of her children were sleeping and the third was cuddling up with Aunt Sally, spooning. The uncle was flat on his back, occasionally rocking himself side to side to distract from his discomfort. The entire clan looked spent but the entire clan was alive to fight another day. Josephine waved us over in a manner that telegraphed she did not intend to be ignored. Squeaky wheels do get the grease.

When a person is against the wall for time, the ones who are quiet are more likely to be passed over, so yes, it is a good idea to speak up. On the other hand, if a person becomes abusive in their requests, there is more of a conscious effort to avoid them. Fortunately, I personally hadn't run across any patient who was demanding in an abrasive way; it just wasn't part of the West African demeanor.

Casper and I went over, hoping this was our last stop and hoping the request would be something easy and quick. Josephine peered up at us through her bloodshot eyes then quietly demanded why the milk promised earlier in the day had not been delivered. I told her I didn't know but that I could go look for some, that often times there were unopened cartons in other buildings with other pediatric patients. Casper and I fanned out and luck was with us, an entire box of a dozen cartons of formula was next door, allowing us to take half and return the conquering heroes. We popped the tabs on a carton, a struggle for a healthy person to pop the waxy tabs without creating a mess, let alone a patient in the grasp of severe fatigue. Josephine took the opened carton and produced a 25cc syringe, expertly drawing up the milk then brushing the nipple of the syringe across the lips of her youngest, agitating the child until she opened her mouth in resignation to take the formula. She did the same for the next oldest and handed the now half empty carton to Sally who poured a bit into a cup that she, too, had to prod the child to drink.

I looked over all of their charts. Everyone had a patent IV, a near miracle in of itself but a good sign, indicating as a lot the Kargbo clan understood the IV's had medical value, thus they helped take care to prevent dislodging them. Everyone continued to run fevers but there were no signs of involuntary diarrhea, everyone dry. More encouraging was the Styrofoam meal containers were neatly stacked and all had at least some of the food missing, hopefully eaten by them and not the dogs, though if the dogs did it I doubt the adults would have taken the bother to care for their impromptu cupboard. I collected up some children's acetaminophen into the droppers, each child getting a weight based dose, Josephine and Sally quietly commanding the children to comply. The uncle was restless with pain and appeared relieved when offered Paracetamol and Valium, washing it all down with about two cups of water, his swallow strong and intact.

It was both impressive and a relief that the Kargbos, as a group, were receptive and involved in their care, understanding the importance of nutrition. Without a doubt, the Major, Jim, Susy and the national nurses were doing an excellent job of teaching the importance of the treatment plan and had everyone on board, making it easier for those that followed up, beating down the odds of a negative outcome. Josephine had a foundational determination and fight, her fear turned into a focused resolve that embraced the weapons of what western medicine had to offer in her family's battle. In many patients, Ebola robbed them of the normal daily concerns over hygiene and appearance, but not the Kargbos, each one dressed and combed, their toothbrushes neatly put away and unworn clothes folded and stacked. I don't know if each tended their own needs, but I strongly suspect that the most well of the family made certain the others were comfortable, that Josephine was the presence no one wished to disappoint.

Casper circled the inside of the building, spraying spots of refuse where he found them while I jotted out a couple of notes on the family. When he returned, I could see the sweat pouring off his brow and into his eyes. No doubt I looked no less different. The two of us had reached our end and needed out, but my fear was once that we stepped through the door there would be another ambulance waiting to unload. It was past 8 p.m., meaning national nurses were off the clock, a scheduling issue that was overlooked when our own schedules were expanded.

We stepped out onto the front walkway; no less than four dogs were tearing into a neglected plastic bag of garbage containing a fair amount of left over patient food. A couple of them looked up at us then resumed their foraging, nipping at one another as they repositioned themselves to take another tear at their find. It used to be dogs ran at the sight of us but now we were just becoming part of the scenery. Or maybe I had it backwards, that they were just becoming part of our scenery, that we were resigned to their being on the grounds once the sun set. Casper, who had no intention of keeping their company, and before I could even think of swearing at the dogs, stepped out ahead of me, adjusted his spray nozzle to stream and let loose with his bleach at the whole of the bunch. The initial reaction of the animals was to freeze, then when they found the distaste and sting of chemicals something to be avoided and feared, they fled at a full run towards the back fence, disappearing into the dark corners the ETU lights didn't reach, Casper filling the shadows of the entire ETU with a cloud of obscenities.

For all of our efforts to minimize the risk of the transfer of the Ebola virus outside the fence, all the spraying, the attention to our gear and the respect for and attention to the unbending protocol of doffing, packs of feral dogs were not of our world, another dimension that we completely rationalized away as being a nonissue. Factually, no one had any hard data or even what I'd call an arguable hypothesis as to why the canine ingress and egress at will was not an infectious disease safety concern. No one knew where these dogs were coming from, other than the general area, or where they were going to, other than the general area. Could anyone even answer the question of what the normal territorial range of a feral dog was in the Port Loko area? Probably not.

At sunrise, people stirred and began their days. For some, that likely meant they would feed the family dog, a sort of quasi pet/master relationship where man and beast claimed no ownership or loyalty to one another, a relationship casual enough that if one or the other suddenly stopped appearing, it was nothing more than a passing thought for the dog on the way to finding another patron, or for the household to tolerate the next dog that moved in. The odds had to be at least a couple of the dogs, of the hundred or so that came in and out of the ETU, were returning to a household during the day, where a person would give them a quick pat and rub, or the kids would hug them, hanging off their backs and necks and getting their faces licked.

Was the distance between here and 'there', wherever 'there' was, sufficient enough that any Ebola virus on the pads of the paws was shed into the dirt, a hostile enough environment that the virus wouldn't survive more than a couple of hours? Probably. The odds of a person walking on a spot where a live virus clung are remote in itself, even then the person would need a break in the skin of the sole of the foot as an entry point. The amount of viral load retained would have to be a large enough inoculating dose, a dose of 10 live virus being the accepted absolute minimum needed for infection, a quantity so inestimably small that the only way to comprehend it is in atomic terms. An entire galactic size count of virus can exist on a pin head if all of Ebola were a universe. The only reasonable reaction is one of astonishment that none of us healthcare workers, cleaners and sprayers had been infected if 10 live virus is indeed size enough for an inoculating dose. What odds that some small stray droplet didn't weave the space between our visors and into our eyes, or survive the doffing process where the tiniest of spots is missed?   More than several cases of infected workers investigated found no known breaches in gear or the disinfecting protocol, meaning that somewhere something wasn't adequately disinfected, and became a touch surface risk. The many different ways we moved about in our environment each day, it was nearly impossible to isolate a specific act. It would be no different trying to track an animal's movements.

The fact that dogs have some sort of natural immunity to Ebola is highly likely, that conclusion gleaned from the fact that no one knew of any cases where a dog suffered from such an infection and succumbed. An animal, human or non-human, can technically be infected by certain organisms but suffer no negative consequences. A common example in humans would be Methecylin Resistant Staph Aureus, MRSA for short. In the United States, about 50% of the population is now technically infected, meaning if we were swabbed nasally or rectally, and that swab cultured in the lab, that sample would yield a result of positive. For people immunocompromised in some way, those being HIV infected, brittle diabetics or recent surgical subjects for instance, they are prime territory for staph infections such as MRSA to bloom and wreak havoc. For the remainder of us, we just live with it. To date, no one has formally studied the possibilities of dogs and Ebola, meaning it cannot be ruled out that dogs can be actively infected, possibly a vector similar to how members of the ape family, including humans in the broad sense, are vectors. Blood tests on dogs in infected regions with active outbreaks reveal dogs to be seropositive, meaning that antibodies to Ebola are detectable. So can Fido transmit? If what we know about the cross transmission of disease between canine and human holds, no, Ebola is not likely transmissible from casual contact such as master feeding or rough housing with the family pet.

If I were outside the fence, and were to spot and know a certain dog was a regular intruder inside the ETU, would I engage him like I might engage some other person's pet, with a rub and pat and a couple of compliments? I'd likely skip the compliments and definitely would skip the friendly touches and deliver a couple of curses, maybe even do a couple of bluff charges in hopes of keeping the dog leery of people in general, hopefully make them think twice about being anywhere people are. Dogs too often find rotting items, such as we find in our own garbage, to be attractive enough to not only eat but to roll in, a sort of canine perfume. I never witnessed an ETU dog rolling in ETU garbage but I have seen them lying down in filth, taking a breather from their dumpster diving.

The fences surrounding the ETU were mostly a visual barrier. It provided the patients with a measure of privacy from the public and a warning about what was in bounds and out of bounds for anyone coming or going. But for the dogs, and possibly one eight year old boy, the fence as something impervious was a moot point, armed soldiers or police notwithstanding. This was a region of the world where shooting dogs en masse was part of disease control, such as in bringing a rabies epidemic to heal, and not uncommon. I was left wondering why the coming and going of the dogs into and out of the ETU was not being addressed at all, even if the only plausible solution was the barrel of a gun, something that would no doubt generate a landslide of negative publicity. Realistically, it could not be dismissed as a reasonable precaution. At end of the day, other concerns were more immediate, and that was to try to save the lives of the infected.

Casper set out for the doffing station but before I followed, I screwed up the courage to look back over into the admissions area. No flashing blue lights, no one standing at the fence trying to wave us over to let us know there was another patient waiting. No sprayers were waiting for us at the doffing station, forcing Casper to yell several times to get someone's attention from inside the sprayers' tent. When someone finally emerged, it was clear Casper had woken them, the sprayer in nightclothes he covered with a winter jacket before donning to spray us down and walk us through the doffing process.

During the time the sprayer took to gear up, I took it as an opportunity to do some house cleaning, picking up some of the many stray nails and left over tin cuttings from the perpetual construction, items just waiting to pierce a boot or gash a suit. The joke about all the nails was that it was a good thing we had our tetanus shots up to date. (And, no, at this point I shouldn't have to explain such a joke.) Eventually, Casper and I were sprayed down, the lack of movement meaning we were no longer generating heat, that our hyper moist condition that helped cool us to comfort was now working too well and causing the both of us to catch the chill out of the night air. By the time we finished, it was nearly 9:00 p.m., meaning the two of us were inside nearly four and a half hours, well beyond the 90-120 minute time limit.

The walk back to the nurses' station was quiet, as quiet as the unit had ever been when I was present, a night and day comparison. I just wanted into some dry clothes and carried an extra pair in my bag every day precisely for that reason. After toweling down and getting a fresh, clean pair of scrubs back on, I began to warm back up enough that a 1.5 liter bottle of ORS water was actually refreshing, something my body sorely needed to fend off the cramps that would come if my experience with hot weather distance running and marathon lawn mowing sessions were at all instructive. After 15 minutes of just sitting and getting my strength back, I noticed I was hungry, but was unable to scare up anything to eat, no big deal since supper would most likely be waiting back at the compound.

Up on the file cabinet top were the binder notebooks with some sort of vague patient chart we were now being asked to fill out when we exited the unit, an utter piece of nonsense that added nothing to what Gwyn's whiteboard in admissions displayed or the patient's bedside chart. There was talk of iPads and a wireless transmission system where we would place the iPads inside, set so they could transmit to devices outside. That meant getting the tablets or laptops, setting up a system, making sure they were routinely charged or powered, a problem in of itself where electrical surges are part of diesel generated electricity, plus keeping the fragile electronics dry and free from corrosive bleach spray. I hoped it wouldn't happen; it would add nothing to what we were able to do.

Charting is an American obsession. I cannot speak for Great Britain, Canada, France or any other nation in the developed world, all who no doubt keep excellent patient records, but when those same health professionals are plugged into the American system, the singular item foreign doctors and nurses comment on is the redundant and voluminous charting Americans engage in, who often times spend the majority of their work days keeping it up to date. At our ETU, that obsession was rearing its hydra headed self, threatening death of morale by a thousand meaningless entries where the job was to treat one diagnosis, that fact alone a blessing which allowed everyone to learn quickly the basics and nuances of the Ebola treatment strategies. In the last 10 days or so, we finally had enough people, managing to get a lab up to speed and seeing some movement towards reliable supply lines for rags, lafas, medications and blankets, covering the essentials for patient care. The video monitoring system being pondered to monitor patients was merely a Rube Goldberg solution to a nonexistent problem that could be solved by simply putting someone outside the fence, at the ready, to receive and relay messages.

Our tendency to complicate matters reminded me of a story about motorcycle manufacturer Harley-Davidson. A multimillion-dollar ceiling system for delivering parts along the assembly line was put into place, but proved complicated and unreliable. The eventual solution to getting the correct parts to workers on the line were simple wooden racks on castors, wheeled down the line as needed.

I detest excess and the superfluous as much as I detest exiguous and scarcity. Tools and resources matter. Just ask any carpenter or mechanic with thousands of dollars in tools how frustrating it is to find you do not have that special tool for specialized items to complete a step that allows one to hasten a task. The same holds true in the world of medicine. Often time a patient's condition may be treated ethically and adequately with a generic medication. Instead, under-patent versions of the same medication, more profitable thanks to patent protection choking off competition from rivals, are prescribed. Too often prescribers are incentivized with money, travel vouchers for hotels and flights and other rewards. The tool, medication, is often essentially the same as an older version but redesigned somewhat more creatively, adding nothing of note to accomplishing treatment goals.

Surgery suites deal with this issue constantly, bombarded with new surgical tools that make high claims of better outcomes, when in fact there has been no real testing to state that conclusion. The DaVinci system, a high end technical robot where the machine's every movement is controlled by the surgeon, was marketed as solving multiple parasurgical problems, promising to lower infection rates, boost patient trust and confidence plus speed recovery times, all worthy goals. Except it doesn't do anything new that high quality tools under an experienced hand already don't do, ranging from specialized eye glasses for detail work to hand rests to help steady the hand to diligent attention to infection prevention strategies perfected over the last century. The 'miracle' of DaVinci is that so many hospitals bought it, paying millions, millions that need to be recovered by employing and charging for it. In the meantime, all the grand claims are bereft of sound, objective data gathered by a disinterested third party. Though recently, I've come across several articles where such studies, not yet complete, are showing that DaVinci is an overpriced scalpel in the hands of a so-so prosthetic hand. One of the unique things about the economics of medicine is that technology has not made patient care cheaper, but has driven costs well above the rate of inflation. It seems the thinking is, 'Why offer a service or product for 100 bucks when you can offer it for 10,000'? Cancer drugs illustrate this conundrum eloquently.

"I think your optimism is healthy," I told her. "But too much optimism can be a bad thing, just like too much pessimism."

She countered me, saying, "No, looking on the bright side of things is never bad."

"Well," I said, "General Custer had a pretty good feeling about Big Horn and the Donner Party about getting across those mountains."

Sneering a slight bit at me, Mary asked, "So what's your point?"

"Excessive optimism can be just as catastrophic as excessive pessimism. One causes people to ignore real risks and the other preventing real improvements."

"And what are we here?" she asked, laying the trap I was more or less willing to walk into.

"Neither. And I mean this: I think we're all pretty much realistic. The only question is, are we ready to quickly correct our errors or defer to not being the squeaky wheel out of fear that we might hurt someone's feelings, maybe make ourselves look like troublemakers."

"Are you going to complain about those?" Mary asked, pointing to the binder in my hands and the mess of papers sprawled across my lap.

"No. The perfect solution is to let this die a natural death. Eventually, we'll figure out that this can be ignored and that it adds nothing."

Mary smiled, nodding her agreement that such unspoken strategies had their place and time. Both of us were tired. She handled the phone the entire night, managing the false starts, misplaced information and unexpected requests that come with trying to plan for something that announces no plan, that being disease and ambulance drivers. Ibrahim was waiting for us outside, bundled in a winter jacket and running the heater on the minivan to keep comfortable. The trip into town was ghostly, the only people out being groups of sketchy looking young men gathered away from any lights. Dogs darted out of ditches, heads down and tails between their legs, on prowl. Dutch camp was well lit and welcoming and Mary asked if I wanted to get a bite and something to drink, knowing that I might not have supper waiting as I was hoping, but the guard at the gate said I wasn't to be allowed in unless I was given a preclearance by the camp director. Ibrahim and I watched Mary walk in, then left to head back to our own beds. He had been working all day since early morning, not only driving people to and from work but making pickup trips of new staff in Freetown.

I looked out the window of the van through the darkness, barely able to make out the Kopa tree where Bernard and his friends gathered for drinks at night. No one was out on the benches and not a single light to be seen. The Ghetto was quiet, past midnight now, so quiet that not even the usual swish of the fruit bat wings plying the air was audible, having finished up their feeding work now that the patio lights were off for the night. No food was out on the table and the freezer inside had no left overs. On the shelf, I found some crackers and left over peanut butter, gobbling just enough to take the edge off my hunger but not sating it. I ignored cleaning up, other than brushing my teeth, and crawled into bed, grateful that the cool nights made sleeping without a fan possible.

Fire Pit

Spending the morning around the compound, waiting to go to work on the evening shift, has its benefits and drawbacks. Like I said earlier, what makes second and third shift less than desirable is you are out of the loop socially, have sleep disruption and are spending your waking hours waiting to go to work all day, a dreading sort of anticipation. At the Ghetto, there was no one else present to help wile away the free time. The electricity was off, so being in the room to read wasn't the most comfortable and the couple of souls that did come and go were themselves working, not having free time to kill for chatting or hitting the market square. I didn't want to kill my book since I had more than two weeks to go thus the next best thing was to wander around the neighborhood and talk up the locals. The adults were nice enough but our language barrier prevented us from truly getting to know each other. However, I learned that a can of cola was a kid magnet, literally bringing them out of their houses and from behind the trees and brush—or at least the brush not burned over in the seasonal fires. I asked them if they missed being in school due to an Ebola emergency order; the answer was a resounding 'no', the kids looking at me as if I had two heads with only half a brain for both. Some things are exactly the same the world over.

During my walk about, it was impossible to ignore the refuse of plastic water bags, food containers, boxes and whatever else no longer had use. Some homes were diligent in placing their garbage in a specific spot until it amounted to being worthwhile to burn, while others were quite comfortable letting something hit the ground, letting nature run its course. Our fire pit outside the north wall of the Ghetto was basically an incident in the ground, an accumulation of plastic water bottles, paper, degraded clothes and discarded food containers. Once a week or so, the house workers would set alight the rubbish and burn it away, smoking shared cigarettes in the orange glow as they watched, the fire an act of hygienic necessity to discourage vermin from settling in, be it insects, rodents or dogs. Tigger found no need to rummage our garbage pile, getting enough to eat that even when offered something off the table like fish or chicken, he would sometimes ignore it.

The day whittled down to my shift's start time and it was as good as a day as any to walk to work, so I took off on foot. Down in the market square on the city center circle, all the shops were up and open again, the merchants trying to recover the lost revenue from the past 3 days of lockdown, a useless attempt at disease control since it was not the market places or places of business where transmission was occurring. I have to confess this is only a hindsight observation and at the time, any idea that could be argued as a good idea was given serious consideration. How could it not. It was common knowledge at the point of the lockdown that the primary environments for transmission of Ebola were within the households where sick relatives and friends cared for each other, where highly personal contact occurs. In the marketplace, people do not make it a practice to conclude a sale by giving a big hug and drinking from the same cup, then giving one another assistance with bathing. When someone is feeling feverish and ill, the only time an Ebola afflicted individual is infectious to others, other than being recently deceased, they tend to stay close to home. It was good to see the markets bustling along again, that life was trying to reach for some sense of normalcy and familiarity, a true position of strength from which to deal with a crisis.

The walk across the Bankasoka river bridge was the usual scene of groups of swimmers, bathers and women beating out laundry. The unfinished power dam continued its mute testament and witness to everything wrong with the politics and finance of third world nations, the mystery of how so much ambition to improve the human condition could evaporate into a sort of an invisible apathy. Motorcycles were again beeping horns to forewarn or say hello, weaving around pedestrians who had loads of plantains or firewood balanced on their head wraps, or the dogs, goats and chickens challenging the traffic. My walk continued with the usual interruptions of shouts of 'Apatow' from the kids and a wave from the Imam sitting on his porch along with other neighbors waving me a good afternoon. It occurred to me I felt less self-conscious of walking through Port Loko than if I were back home, where walking can be considered an unusual and suspicious enough activity that people call the police to report it. After all, back in the States, normal people drive a car everywhere except in walking cities like New York or Washington D.C. It's only the odd duck you see walking down the road.

Soon enough I was at Maforki, everyone busy at work. It was a good time to take the extra ten minutes to catch my breath and relax before diving into the evening shift duties. The nurses' station was empty, all the staff probably at meetings or in the hot zone finishing the afternoon round. All the workers were back at it, still minus George who had not been released as promised, a troubling sign that either something was done to him or that management and government was using his imprisonment as a warning to the others should they get any ideas to reenact the previous protests. With nothing to do in the nurses' station, I wandered outside and over to the fence to kill some minutes, just watching how it all worked.

In the hot zone, cleaners were carrying out the full slop buckets over to a makeshift latrine area, emptying them and bringing them back to the courtyard to wash, laying them out to sun dry. Other cleaners were taking the plastic garbage cans and emptying them into even larger cans that were dumped into black plastic garbage bags that were then doubled up and double tied. After two of the bags were filled, a cleaner would carry the bags over to the fire pit and toss them in, ensuring a near continuous smell of smoldering wet clothes, old food and medical waste over and through the compound. There were never roaring flames and the cleaners would prod the piles in the pit with long sticks, stirring it to let the coals breathe and heat up enough to burn away what they fed into the pit. Anyone old enough to remember the American landfills prior to the mid 70's recognizes immediately the acrid smell of burning garbage. Before I even saw the fire pit, I could smell it and knew how Maforki's garbage was being handled.

Nolan was on his phone and laptop simultaneously, conducting the daily symphony of making sure who was getting where when and that every possible hurdle was being lowered enough to clear. As soon as one phone call ceased, another began, an endless stream of items and ideas getting organized by sheer force of his will and personality, turning on the charm as needed and pulling out the minor threats when all else was failing. The new fire pit was not in use as far as I knew, but here I was looking at it and it was the conclusion of one of Nolan's multi marathon series of phone calls that ended getting it built, meaning it was he who secured the money, found the carpenters, found the materials and managed the time lines. It was a small project by American standards, something a couple of buddies would do in their spare time back in the states but over here it was a formidable undertaking that required diligence and a knowing how to find what you needed fast in a place that was literally foreign. Even finding nails was an all day affair since there were no central building suppliers, no big box store where Nolan could one stop shop for fire pit materials. A Menard's would have been more than handy.

Back and forth the cleaners went with the bags of refuse, handling them by holding them away from their bodies so that a stray needle might not accidentally poke through the bags, their own hazmat suits and through their own skin, something that would be considered a high risk breach and get them thrown into quarantine. For someone like me or my expat colleagues, such a breach would be a one way ticket home, a million dollar plane ride, landing us in one of the four centers set up throughout the United States to handle high-risk suspect Ebola patients. For those like the cleaners or national nurses or sprayers, such a breach would land them most likely in Kerrytown at a hospital not nearly as well equipped and certainly not as materially comfortable as what was in Bethesda or Nebraska or even close to what the US Army had erected in Liberia. The double standard was unsettling to think about and it certainly was never spoken of openly that I heard. It made me sad and was a genuine slap of reality of how unfair or unequal the world is, be it by intent or accident.

I would be alarmed and concerned if one of my fellow workers came down ill, or so I thought. I was disabused of that notion when a national nurse we worked with reported as being ill. However, the name and circumstances of the possible cause was kept from us, other than to say she was presenting with Ebola like symptoms that were eventually confirmed as Ebola. Without a face or name, unable to know what personal connection there was, she was anonymous and invisible, an event of *something* that happened, not *someone* who needed our support by emotion or even medicine. 'It' became a faceless casualty.

As horrible as the old Soviet Stalin regime was under that mass murderer, he spoke at least one remarkably sad truth: "The death of one man is a tragedy, the death of millions is just a statistic." The meaning is that we can empathize with the travails of one man when we know enough about that man to relate a personal understanding. But for a million it is anonymous, just too much to comprehend or not enough to understand. Thinking about it is enough to make a person question the depths of their humanity, making it a topic to be avoided even in private personal reflection. For soldiers who are unable 'turn it off', they have nightmares, night sweats and general anxiety disorders. For anyone else who encounters death or despair as part of their jobs, they, too, must learn to 'turn it off'. Those that can't often began to self implode. Worse, they began to deteriorate in ways which openly dehumanize those they are entrusted to protect. There is nothing more vulnerable than a person in a desperate situation who has no means of coping, be it emotionally, financially or socially. They may find themselves forced to trust a person with power. For the twisted, dented protectors this can be blood in the water, a chance to use the power of the club or the power of knowledge to manipulate a situation to be even more deranged for the already harmed.

The psychology of response to large disasters, socially and individually, is difficult to pin down but one study by a fellow named Slovic offers some insight:

"Slovic asked people to imagine they were disbursing money on behalf of a large foundation: They could give $10 million to fight a disease that claimed 20,000 lives a year -- and save 10,000 of those lives. But they could also devote the $10 million to fight a disease that claimed 290,000 lives a year -- and this investment would save 20,000 lives.

Slovic found that people preferred to spend the money saving the 10,000 lives in the first scenario rather than the 20,000 lives in the second scenario: "People were responding not to the number of lives saved but the percentage of lives saved. In the one case, their investment could save half the victims; in the case of the more deadly disease, it could save 7 percent of the victims," he said. (http://reason.com/blog/2009/01/07/the-death-of-one-man-is-a-trag)

Per the above, we respond to proportions, supporting my hypothesis, and Stalin's, that large numbers are too much to ingest emotionally. It casts a pall like you're inside a mausoleum, a moss creeping over your skin, to think about the cold calculus of it all.

But back to the infected colleague. I never learned the name and never found out if they lived or died, though I assume they survived since no bad news ever made it back to me. Becoming infected was an occupational hazard we all worked with and accepted and respected, but no one feared. Knowledge is the antidote that allows us to critically consider the value of risks vs rewards and face events that, at first blush, appear to be dangerous or life threatening. Tested and established routines performed with mindfulness allowed us Ebola workers to navigate patient care without being overwhelmed by concerns for our own safety. This is like the skydiver who learns how to read an altimeter and manage their gear that allows them to enjoy the exhilaration of freefall without being terrorized by the possibility of smashing into a cornfield at 130 mph. Most of all, you learn to trust your tools, your own judgment and your colleagues. I fully trusted that if I, or one of my cohorts became ill, we would be given adequate care with resources above and beyond what we were able to provide for our own patients, a stark illustration of being a 'have' versus my patients who were 'have nots', something that tends to gnaw at a me a bit.

Nolan put away his laptop and phone and let his frame slump in the chair, the anxiety of deadlines withering away and dripping out of his fingertips. Visibly, I could see he was actually catching his breath.

"Everything getting done?" I asked, attempting to commiserate.

"Today? Yes. For once, it's all OK." Then he looked at me, simultaneously smiling and soliciting, to say, "You have no idea how hard it is to keep you people fed and watered."

"Jesus, Nolan," I teased, "You make it sound like you're running an animal shelter."

"Hey, it sort of is. Had to make sure all of you had your papers and shots..."

Before he could extend the simile, the nurse's station was hit by a sudden "KawWumph!" The building's framing shook enough that the slack of the tarped walls made a sharp sounding 'crack!' like a wet towel being whipped and snapped. We both jumped to our feet with me saying, "I know that sound. It's the sound of gasoline fumes igniting."

Out the door and down the covered concrete walk we went. For those outside, no one seemed alarmed or even all that curious, pretty much every one concluding that it was a fire being lit with petrol, a common enough occurrence that it was something in passing. For Nolan and me, this was a sound of someone maybe being harmed. We arrived at the back of the unit near the showers where the tarp fence separated the hot zone with the fire pits from the rest of the grounds. Ali joined us at the fence just in time to see a black mushroom cloud disintegrate into the sky. The new fire pit was now christened in flame, enough fire that it was licking the tin roof ceiling and wrapping out and around the drip line. It was obvious too much fuel was used to ignite the new pit and that there was too much flammable waste that would continue to feed high flames, burning away the roof trussing and rafters.

Nolan's project was literally going up in smoke, forcing him to concede that it was a matter of minutes before it would be a total loss. Shaking his head in disgust and muttering, he cursed, "That dumb shit. Only an idiot puts gasoline in hole and throws a match to it. Goddamn it!"

Inside the unit but a safe distance away, the cleaner who poured the fuel and threw the match sported wisps of black soot on his white PPE, indicating that he was likely leaning over into the pit when he threw the match that exploded the gas fumes, close enough to get a blast of fire and singed air.

"Are you alright?" Nolan shouted to the cleaner. The cleaner nodded back that he was.

Nolan, unable to contain his anger, erupted at the cleaner, shouting, "Listen you dumb ass Wile E Coyote. You don't use gasoline in a hole to start a fire. You're lucky you don't have that suit melted into your skin."

The sheepish body language of the cleaner relayed that he understood his screw up. Ali looked at the cleaner and shook his head, shouting some sort of insult in Temne at the man that made the cleaner's shame even more pronounced in his body language. Ali turned to Nolan and me and asked, "Are there people in America who embarrass their countrymen as he shames mine?", pointing to the cleaner who was standing still, not sure if he should come out of the unit or keep watch over his act of arson.

Nolan, finding the opportunity for humor in the tragic, answered, "Yes. But we keep them all under a dome in one place—Washington D.C."

Ali looked at his feet, thinking, then looked back up at Nolan, naively and seriously asking, "You put all your village fools in the capital city?"

Nolan continued his explanation, adding, "We put a lot of them on TV, too."

I laughed, but the reference was lost on Ali, who decided there was something he wouldn't understand so kept his quiet.

Meanwhile, the flames pulled back some but continued to reach up out of the pit far enough to lick at the wooden frame, sparks and embers visible as the frayed shavings of the lumber reached their ignition point and turned a bright orange-red. Some of the lumber was turning black with white ash spotting it, evidence that heat was taking its toll. After a few more minutes, the lumber began to sprout flames here and there and finally turned into red hot coals that were too weak to hold up the tin roof and its own frame. First, a cross member would sag then a another would follow, followed further by a corner support twisting out and bringing the rafters down low enough for the burning waste to ignite them. The tin roof panels reacted with a popping metallic sound as they creased from the heat and eventually oxidized into a dull gray-black. After 15 minutes, one end of the roof fell into the pit, shunting the heat and flame to the other end that quickly worked to knock out the remaining support, collapsing the roof down to the ground to cover the pit before folding on itself and falling in.

Nolan became philosophical, letting his natural inclination to optimism brighten up a sad situation. "Hey, at least we have a spare fire pit. And Larry, Curly, Moe is lucky he's in anonymous PPE."

The afternoon call to prayer came and Ali headed towards the prayer room, telling Nolan he'd pray for Allah to deliver him a new fire pit. Nolan looked at Ali and smiled, telling Ali that maybe he should pray that the cleaner gets to keep his job once Dr. George would found out that he burned Maforki's new fire pit to the ground.

I find it all ironic. We burned a fire pit burn to the ground. The cleaner set around the backside of the Confirmed buildings and disappeared. Several others came up to survey the damage and left, no doubt able to pin the finger on the culprit. My guess was that in the current climate over work issues amongst the nationals, they were reluctant to out the fellow, my hope being that he would indeed keep his job, a job that was very likely supporting an entire extended family. My shift hadn't even started; already it was shaping up to be a challenge.

The Strangulation of Reason

The fire pit incident went viral. Dr. George knew. He was heading out for the day on his way to the government hospital when we bumped into each other. I asked if there was going to be a response such as letting go the cleaner and building a new fire pit cover. He smiled and shook his head, saying, "It is moments like this we need to have a little whiskey. No one is to blame under these circumstances." I was happy to hear his empathy and that the cleaner was in no danger of forfeiting his work.

Outside the front fence, the radio blared BBC world updates and news coverage from Europe and Africa. The admissions building had a small group milling about the shade, survivors and family of survivors. Our little tree was running out of room on its branches to have more ribbons tied to its smooth, chocolate bark and Africa green leaves subdued by the reds, yellows and blues of the ribbons cut from lafas, shirts or dresses of the survivors. Someone put a ring of poured, formed cement around the base of the tree and various persons pressed their names into the wet cement before it dried to concrete. One scribble I noticed was that someone had etched in 'PCR −', a reference to a discharged survivor's laboratory status, a sort of inside joke.

Each survivor, both middle aged women, held up their Certificate of Cure issued by the Sierra Leone government for photographs taken by family cell phones and staff cameras. Several Cubans had come over to pose with the survivors, their smiles as wide and bright as the family members that greeted the discharged patients. The van driver was becoming visibly impatient, pacing around the door of the van, anxious to get on his way since at least one family lived a good 80 kilometers out and, likely, part of the trip involved car-swallowing dirt roads. With their new bedding, cooking oil, rice and cash, the group settled in and headed east down the highway, the first stop being the Total gas station for petrol and maybe for the survivors to spend part of their discharge cash on a rare treat of Coca-Cola.

With day shift winding up their duties and preparing to head home, I headed into the admissions building to take notes off the board and catch up with who went where when. Gwyn and Musa were working their phones, focused on whatever task was in front of them. Jabari sat on the bench against the wall under one of the two large open air windows, his chin resting on his chest, no doubt napping. Two phlebotomists poured over the admissions books to discern how many blood draws they needed to do and on whom, comparing it to the names on the whiteboard of those previously admitted into Suspect or moved to Confirmed. The tension was less palatable the last few days now that systems were in place and the kinks ironed out, even though we were busier. But a new sort of anxiety was settling in, that being able to keep up with the sheer number of new cases.

The DERC and NERC reports continued to show a steady climb in new Ebola cases. Our Port Loko district was now open 24 hours a day to receive anyone who arrived by foot or ambulance who met the criteria of fever and contact with an infected person(s). There was room enough inside to accommodate the burgeoning patient load but the challenge was having enough staff to adequately address patient needs around the clock. Day shift was well covered but evening shift was two of us alone with a national nurse until 8 p.m. After that hour, I either had to stay out or, at the very minimum, have a sprayer trail me. Mary was still out of action until her cut cleared up but that was a positive since she could handle the phone, start up the paper work and put together the patient's admission bucket, bedding and initial medications.

I pulled up next to Jabari on the bench, absent-mindedly shuffling my tennis shoes through the red dirt while I piled up my PPE gear neatly to be ready to go for when I had to handle the first admission. Gwyn was going over phone numbers of various contacts we might have to solicit from Catholic Charities orphanage to Port Loko social services and the assorted ambulances, doctors and other information. Jabari was now in full slump, softly snoring away under the late afternoon heat.

Gwyn whirled around a few more times between copy machines, file cabinets and phone calls but then corralled Mary and I to her desk, going over the twenty odd new admissions so far that day and bringing our attention to a list of potential admissions, five so far, that would likely be coming in from the outlying areas of the Port Loko district. By all accounts, we wouldn't see our first admission for at least another two hours, sometime between supper and dusk. In the meantime, there was at least one discharge that could be brought to the fence, meaning I was going to suit up earlier than wanted. My thinking was that it was only one so it should be quick enough to allow me back out to take a break and eat before having to gear back up and take care of the later admissions. The optimism of my plan was about to be tested in a way I should have anticipated enough to fortify myself with food and water. I was about to pay for that miscalculation.

Gwyn packed her bag and ended her day, leaving the evening shift skeleton crew to fend for itself. Jabari stirred and I brought him up to the minute about the day's one final discharge, a boy of 14 whose lab result was temporarily misplaced, delaying his going home. Jabari offered to run the fence with clothes and anything else I might need, a decent gesture that would keep him at work later than he needed to be. His constant upbeat attitude was good for morale so I didn't feel too guilty about not insisting he go home for the night. For Jabari, Sierra Leone was indeed still home even though he was now an American citizen of nearly a decade, back here in the crisis fulfilling his sense of obligation and duty to his country of birth as best he could.

Joseph was the sprayer I wrangled up, a young man who looked like he could still be in the middle grades. I tested our communication abilities between the two of us and found they were not great but adequate enough. No national nurses were available, either having gone home or were involved in the supper meal. No matter. All simple enough.

Joseph and I went in and began our search for Imatu Kargbo, 14 year old male in Confirmed 3. Upon entering Confirmed 3, it was obvious everyone inside was in no shape to go anywhere, all obviously ill and nowhere near being recovered. Nonetheless, we went person to person reading wrist bands and repeating Isatu Kargbo's name, hoping to elicit some direction to his whereabouts. Nothing.

We exited the Confirmed 3 and hopped on over to Confirmed 4 and went through the same routine of checking wristbands and soliciting for clues with no luck. Next on down was Confirmed One and Two, only to come up empty handed. Jabari watched all this from the fence and figured out our problem, calling us over to give us some direction.

"You can't find him, right?" Jabari smiled through his laugh.

"Nope. Don't tell me he's been discharged already and that we're on a wild goose chase," I half pleaded.

"Oh, no," Jabari laughed. "That would be easy."

"What?"

Jabari shook his head, bemused, then filled Joseph and me in on what was happening. "Isatu heard he was being discharged and thought he'd help us along so he moved back over to Suspect Two where he first came into. Apparently he figured that going home meant he would be retracing his steps through the ETU."

"How do you know this?" I asked.

Jabari pointed over to the front deck of Suspect 2. "That's probably him. He has everything packed and ready to go it looks like. He's just waiting for you to figure it all out."

This screwed us up. We are never supposed to backtrack from Confirmed back into Suspect, a hard rule to prevent people from going from a known contaminated area into one that theoretically may be contaminated. An infection precaution. This meant Joseph and I would have to go back through the doffing station, decontaminate, then go back through the donning process before being able to go into Suspect and bring Isatu out. What should have taken 30 minutes now was going to stretch out to well over an hour.

We went through the doffing station, back out and around to the admissions building. When we arrived, Jabari was there to greet us, laughing harder than usual. "You're not going to believe this, but he saw you guys and went back over to Confirmed. He's waiting for you there."

"Are you f*** serious?" I yelled. Exasperated, I asked Jabari to make sure Isatu didn't travel back into Suspect before we got to him. Me and Joseph and I donned our gear while Jabari yelled out instructions over the fence to Isatu to not wander back into Suspect. Isatu, not able to hear clearly, started towards the gate that separated the Confirmed and Suspect, causing everyone at the fence to yell out in unison to stay where he was. Isatu's hand rested on the gate, hesitating, then our sprayer yelled again, prompting Isatu to interpret that as a reason to come back into Suspect. Everyone groaned.

Mary offered that it was fine. Since we hadn't headed back in yet we could just escort Isatu to the shower and discharge him from there. True. The only issue was the travel back and forth between Suspect and Confirmed, raising a contamination issue but in reality Suspect was as infected as Confirmed, the only difference being was that in Suspect we didn't yet know for certain who was or wasn't infected.

Joseph pumped his backpack sprayer several times and hit my boots and gloves with a quick dose, the smell of chlorine hitting my nostrils as if a blender went off in my sinuses. Without doubt, the mixture was exceedingly strong. On one hand, it inspires faith that the virus will be killed but on the other, the vapors irritate the throat and should the juice get between your gloves and skin, leave you burned. It's not an accident that chlorine gas is used as a chemical weapon, a blistering agent similar to mustard gas in some respects.

We cracked the gate and met Isatu half way across the courtyard. Joseph translated my instructions to Isatu about bathing and changing out clothes and that Jabari would meet him at the west gate to take him up front to the admissions building for his parting discharge gifts of food and cash. Isatu nodded his understanding and took off on a half run to the faucet. By the time I caught up, he was underneath and soaping up. I think "excited" would be the word.

At the gate, Jabari prodded Isatu to drop the après bath lafa and try out the clothes he picked out of the donated pile of clothes he made his best guess at for size. The jeans looked clean and neat and once on fit better than if Isatu had picked them out himself. The shirt was a royal navy blue and orange, Chicago Bears colors, and sported a Chicago

Bears "C".

I pointed at the orange "C" and shouted, "Bears suck! Go Packers!"

Isatu looked back at me, slightly anxious that maybe he had done something to offend me. Picking up on this, I asked Joseph to tell him it was OK, that he'd done nothing wrong and that it wasn't his fault the Bears couldn't sell their gear, more or less forcing them to give it away. I went on to explain that the Bears were the arch rival of the Green Bay Packers, the home team of where I came from, like Sierra Leone and Liberia were in soccer. Isatu nodded an understanding and smiled, pointing at the "C" on his shirt, "Bears suck." I gave him the thumbs up and out the gate he went. Alive. A bit brainwashed by some of my own hometown propaganda maybe but definitely alive.

"Well, Joseph, give us a pump and spray and let's go catch some supper," I said, looking forward to some fish and vegetables. As we rounded the shower building corner, I could see out across the yard the large front gate being swung open, then the flash of blue light of an ambulance. The first inclination was to swear but it could be a nice surprise, meaning we could take care of the admission now instead of having it interrupt us in the middle of supper. The heat was tolerable, a dry 80 degrees, so being in PPE wasn't oppressive and, at moments, one could feel quite safe and snug in gear like a bear wrapped in a warm winter den, the outside world's worries and scares locked out and away.

Joseph nearly danced over to the ambulance while I paced in step behind him. He told me this would be his first time getting someone out of the ambulance and asked for instruction on what to do, which I did by filling him on how to spray the doors, then open the rear doors so I could look in, then let the patient walk out if they could, and to spray wherever the patient touched or stepped until they took a chair beneath the canopy. If they couldn't ambulate, I'd go in and get them out with an assist or have them stay on the gurney and go through the admission's process that way, then gurney them over to a room. Joseph would spray down the inside of the ambulance once we had the patient out.

The driver was yelling at Josephine and she gave it back as good as he was giving it, loud and excited. I had no idea what they were shouting at each other. I learned over time that the near frantic animated conversations the locals engaged in were of about as much consequence as the polite chit-chat two strangers on an elevator in America had. The driver stayed put, occasionally pounding his hand on the door, which in turn prompted Josephine to run up the fence line and yell back at him. He'd throw up his hand and she'd return to filling out the paperwork.

Joseph waited for my permission to open the rear door. I gave him the OK and he tugged it to the side, the metal hinges sticky from corrosion due to all the sprayed on chlorine. The door stayed open on its own. In the shadow of the patient hold, one man was sitting on the metal bench, his legs propped up on the gurney and his arms crossing his chest. He looked at me and I waved him out. He moved under his own power, stepping off the rear of the ambulance with no stumbles and took a chair beneath the admissions canopy.

Mary and Josephine launched into the questionnaire, asking the 30 year old or so fellow what chiefdom and village he hailed from, his name, birthday and age. I ran the thermometer's red dot across his forehead and came up with 38.5 C, or about 101.4 F. Josephine handed a bottle of water over the fence and I motioned for him to drink, which he did, taking about a third of it down with no problem. We noted his red eyes but clear gums and he reported only a slight headache along with generalized achiness. More questions revealed he was part of a burial team for a relative who was sick for several days before passing away, and that there were rumors of secret burials of Ebola victims in his village to hide the fact and avoid the quarantines and stigma that would come with such open acknowledgement.

"So what made you come here?" Mary asked.

He looked at Mary, quiet, trying to contain his emotions that were so close to the surface. Then a tear broke and he wiped it back, saying, "I don't want to die."

The four of us stared at him, sympathetic, while he put his eyes back to the ground to vale his tears. I put a hand on his shoulder.

"You're not going to die," Mary half ordered, half encouraged the man. "We've become very good at getting people home. Take the medicine and drink the water we give you and you *will* be walking out of here.

Drink some more water."

He put the bottle to his lips and drank another third of the 1.5 liter bottle. Josephine explained the IV needle and why it was important. He surrendered his arm, obvious and easy veins on the dorsal aspect that made the task much easier, though the heavy glue of the IV tape still managed to tenaciously cling to my gloves, prompting another dramatic event where I had to slowly peel away the tape off the surgical glove fingertips without tearing them open, something that should it happen would immediately send me to the doffing station to decontaminate and gear back up to come in and finish the job.

I burrowed into a nightcrawler-sized vein without making a bloody mess or tearing my gloves open. Joseph took over the admission bucket and blankets for the fellow, the items Mary had set on our side of the fence. After getting him to take some Paracetamol and Cipro, I followed it up with 10 mg of oral Valium to help him relax for what was going to be a stressful first night as he adjusted to his struggle. Joseph and I walked him over to Suspect to a dry ward, one where the other patients were quiet and not visibly agonizing, hoping to keep him as calm as could be possible. Inside, he took a clean mattress on the floor in the corner and quickly settled in, using his blanket as a pillow. It was clean. So far. Tomorrow morning it could just as well be a fecal and vomit explosion with overflowing buckets of waste. For now, it was dry and quiet and most important, humane.

Joseph and I walked down the concrete ramp, ready to doff, dry and get some supper. The ambulance had already left but before we could turn through the yard and out, Mary was at the fence waving us back, only to tell us that another ambulance was outside waiting to get through the gates. I swore a little and Joseph looked at me for what to do.

"Are you OK enough to do another one?" I asked, half pleading for him not to abandon me even though he was perfectly within his rights of self-preservation to do so.

Stretching out his all of wiry 5-foot frame, Joseph manned up, saying, "I am strong to go all night." And he meant it.

"Real tough guy," I teased back. "Good. Because I might not be." As I said this, I could feel my socks heavy enough in sweat to fall to my ankles, my toes swimming in the wrinkles of cotton at the end of my boot. There wasn't a dry spot left on me except for my tongue. It was getting dark. Supper was long gone.

Back across the courtyard we went. No moon in the sky and the solar lights were coming on one by one, the soft visual purple of the LED's carving a space out from the encroaching darkness. Out in the center of the courtyard, I stopped to take a breath, listening to the rhythmic labor of my lungs at work. As I tilted my head back to open my throat up to the cool air I was trying to force through my mask, I opened my eyes to see the sky above. Stars. Finally a clear night. The red dust was thin or gone and the stars were scattered like glitter and flecks of silver against a sapphire heavy into dusk. No city lights to crowd them out. Then the last of the courtyard lights flickered and began their graveyard shift work. Rest time over. I put my head down and ahead, focused on Joseph's back, and caught him at the ambulance that was waiting for us.

Josephine had stayed beyond what she needed to be doing, apparently finding it entertaining to argue with the ambulance drivers as she was again immersed in loud, animated discussion. Out of their swells of verbiage, I managed to discern that he had driven over 100 kilometers to get here ,no doubt hoping to get on his way home as quickly as possible. Hey, weren't we all?

Joseph, his spray pack still half full with several gallons, had one strap, tied together with frayed binder twine, slouching off his left shoulder, trying to give his shoulders a rest from the constant tension. Mary's limp was magnified by her constant running in and out of the admission's building for papers, syringes, wrist bands, colored markers and…. Well, it was half the office in her hands and she was glued to the phone at the same time. I pointed at the rear doors of the ambulance and stepped forward after Joseph sprayed them down.

"Are you ready?" Joseph asked, his hand on the latch.

It wasn't like some rabid psycho killer was going to leap out of the back and try to tear my heart out of my chest I thought. The worst it could be was someone with Ebola. There's a joke in there somewhere but I was too tired to arrange it.

"Sure. Go ahead. Open the door," I encouraged.

Joseph uncorked the latch and swung the door wide. I couldn't see anything so I yelled at Josephine to yell at the driver to turn on the cabin light. After a very long and animated conversation, Josephine finally translated back to me, saying, "What is a 'cabin light'?"

I shook my head. "Never mind. Someone get me a flashlight. Remember, it has to be one we can leave in here."

Josephine and Mary went hunting for a flashlight. Joseph in the meantime swung open the second door but that did little to illuminate the setting inside the cabin of the ambulance. He then ordered me to spread and show my hands for a spray down. I could feel the coolness of the spray through my suit and the burst of energy it gave back to me. Then I stepped to the bumper and strained to see as best I could under the low light conditions. There was the gurney and its white sheets. The gurney was empty. The plane of the white metal bench was uninterrupted, meaning nothing or no one was on it.

I shouted to the ambulance driver, "Where's the patient? There's no patient in here." He understood me and from the safety of the cab, shouted back that there was a patient. I jumped up on the rear bumper, placed a knee on the gurney, and leaned in, trying to see. Meanwhile on the other side of the fence, the two women were yelling to me that they couldn't find a flashlight that could go inside. "Figures," I muttered. I crawled to the end of the gurney and then stopped. Suddenly what I was looking for I found with my ears. I couldn't see the patient but I could hear him gurgling. A realization snapped into my mind—death rattle, the sound of a patient with terminal secretions that occurs during the dying process, the throat flooded with fluid that audibly quivered with each inhalation and exhalation. Very unlikely he was conscious.

Where was he? I felt around with my hands against the back and side walls, thinking he would be sitting up but chided myself after realizing that someone with a death rattle was most likely not going to be sitting up. That would be a medical oddity worth mention at the next meeting. I continued feeling around on the floor and then on the left side of the gurney, a more than large enough space for a full grown adult. Nothing but hard metal floor. My eyes were finally adjusting to the darkness and I was able to make out better what surrounded me. Then, to my right, there it was-- the dark shape of an arm breaking the flat pattern of the white sheet. I put my hand on its hand. I squeezed. It didn't squeeze back. I followed the arm down with my hand where it was stopped by the metal side rail of the gurney. I hesitated to force my hand, fearing a tear to a glove or worse, cut myself. Slowly, I pushed my hand forward and kept on alert for pinches or pokes of metal. Eventually I found a shoulder and from there was able to follow up to the man's face. My hand slid effortlessly over the contours of his lips and nose, lubricated by his secretions. Enough.

I crawled back to the door end of the gurney for a better view and could see that the space between the gurney and the metal side bench was all maybe 6 inches, about the length of a dollar bill. I placed my outstretched hand, a length of 7 inches from wrist to fingertip, on the gurney rail and toward the edge of the metal bench figured there was about ½ inch to inch to spare. No way could a man cram into that space I thought.

I crawled back out not to cheers and greetings but admonitions that another ambulance was already outside and waiting for this one to clear. Everyone wanted to know how long it would be before I would be done.

"I have to find him first," I shot back, annoyed at the demand that I should hurry.

"What?" Mary asked. "You can't find the patient?"

"I have him but I have to pull the gurney out and Joe and I have to roll him onto a litter," I instructed. Then looking at Mary and Josephine, I continued, saying, "He won't be able to answer any questions and he isn't going to be able to take any his meds by mouth. He's unconscious. Likely in a coma."

This set Mary and Josephine in motion to start interrogating the ambulance driver for information on the man's name, age and any other personal and medical information he might have with him. I could tell by the tenor of the discussion that they were coming up mostly empty handed. It was bad enough we had someone this critical but it was worse he might be anonymous critical. I turned my attention back to Joseph, who sprayed me down yet once again, and then focused on clearing the cabin so the two of us could get the patient out and into a

side bench. I kept pulling hard. Now his head was up and his torso was coming through tight. At one point, he stopped breathing and moaning, meaning I had him wedged tight enough to halt his ability to fill his inhale. I hastened my muscles to see it through, my biceps, back and shoulders burning from the exertion, my mind closed to the suffering I was inflicting. With a jolt of adrenaline, I yanked again and his chest followed, an audible crepitus as the tension of rib cartilage was rearranged in tiny snaps and crackles. He resumed breathing, the rattle as pronounced as ever but no moan.

I rested on my knees then resolved to finish the job. His hips came through with some resistance but that had to do with his pants getting caught and coming off as I peeled him out of his trousers, bottom half disrobed, and finally got his legs through one at a time and onto the body bag. Done. I stopped myself and focused on arranging the patient for the trip out.

My legs ached, twinges of cramps plucking my calves and thighs, my lungs craving air so much that I had to grip my hand to the gurney rail so I wouldn't paw at my mask. Soon enough the fire left my lungs and bones and I was able to step back outside, letting Joseph cool me off with the chlorine as I sat on the end of the gurney.

Joseph came inside and across from me. "He has no pants."

"They're down in between," I pointed.

He leaned over and reached down and fished out the trousers, laying them on top to restore some dignity I managed to strip from our difficult patient. I thanked Joseph. He was tired but he was still being kind.

We slid the cargo of the man forward and stepped off the bumper, each of us grasping a handle at the head and foot. Steadying ourselves, we pulled the patient the rest of the way out until his full weight bent our knees enough we had to lower him to the ground. Mary and Josephine reminded us to get his temperature and a verbal on the man's medical status. He was in a coma, had a death rattle, dry caked blood around his lips and fouled himself, something Joseph pointed out to me with the fecal brown streaks and smears on my apron, arms and hands when he ordered me to spread for the spray down. Joseph took the wristband

and read off a name that went in my one ear and out the other, my only care being that he wasn't anonymous at least. I decided it was worth placing an IV on the off chance the patient had even a small chance. He was owed at least that for everything he endured. It was decided that I should give 10 mg of valium but there was no IV or IM Valium to give so two pills placed rectally had to suffice, my finger breaching the sphincter with little resistance and only 2 millimeters of surgical glove between my body and a vault full of Ebola. The putrid cess showed some taint of dark blood, suggesting a GI bleed further up. Other than carrying him to a bed, the hardest was over. The moaning had stopped but the rattle continued.

Both of us sat on the ground, our hands in our laps, summing up the strength for the carry-over to Suspect. Finally, the two of us got up, grabbed the bag and began the 65 steps walk over, a number I counted and that has stuck with me. Sixty-five steps from the admission canopy to Suspect 3. I imagined it was a contest and Joseph seemed bent on impressing someone. His small size would have you think he wasn't capable but he more than made up for it with grim determination. What other kind of determination would he have here?

Inside Suspect 3, we stepped over the concrete stoop with our wet cargo. None of the other patients stirred under the garish fluorescent lighting that already did mottled complexions no favors. An empty mattress was on the floor near the rear of the room by a window where we could hang the IV. The first liter ran wide open and was mostly in, so I discarded the bag and threw up the second liter after digging in a pile underneath the meds table, itself a mess where old infant formula and children's sweetened liquid acetaminophen was spilled or left half empty and open, attracting steady lines of tiny red ants. All the effort to make inventory orderly was being ignored, reducing us to hunt and peck and waste valuable time. I found myself frustrated that everyone here who used these tables was organized enough to get through medical training of one sort or another but they couldn't be bothered to put something back where it belonged. It was a disregard for Dr. Galleo's and Francie's work to make all of our jobs better by taking the initiative to build med boxes out of their own wallets.

I found a place on the window frame for the IV bag as well as the patient bedside chart sheet and a clipboard. Down the list of signs and symptoms I went, creating a grim checklist that added up to 'too late'. While I was doing the charting, Joseph was struggling with the man's pants. I almost stopped him, reasoning that they were too fouled but checked myself and helped dress the poor soul. We then propped him up on his side so that any secretions could drain and that he would not asphyxiate on his own snot.

Outside, yet another ambulance was waiting to drop someone into the maw of the camp. Was it really a hospital anymore? The word 'camp' has too many depressing connotations of brutal historical events, camps designed specifically to strip people of dignity and worth. I promised myself that I would never use the word here again.

Josephine and Mary were already pelting the driver with questions and actually getting good information back, enough so that much of the paper work was finished, leaving only the medical assessment for me to do.

At the fence, I rested my arms on my knees then sat down in one of the chairs to rest my feet. My entire body was swimming inside the PPE and my breathing was taking effort to get good inhalations through my mask slopped with my own secretions. I was going to have my own death rattle pretty soon, I thought, if the mask became any more wet. Then Mary put me back to work.

"According the ambulance driver, this guy was found in a village acting strange. There was no known contact with Ebola victims and there isn't any information on his temp or anything else indicating he should be here." Mary flipped over a page, continuing, "By all accounts he is able to speak but doesn't answer questions. He understands English but responds only in Krio or Temne. What do you think?"

I stared at her, shifting foot to foot. "Then why is he being sent to us? You said no temperature and no reported contact with known Ebola victims?"

Mary gave a shrug of being uncertain, saying, "That's the report the ambulance driver gave us. Maybe we can at least get a temperature off him that justifies him being admitted. Otherwise, he can't be dropped here."

I shook my head in confusion, thinking aloud, "Yeah, it doesn't really add up. I'll scan him and see what we have."

Meanwhile, Josephine was again interrogating the ambulance driver for additional information and reported back to us, saying, "The people in the village were scared of the man so they called the ambulance to pick him up. They tried to get his temperature but he refused. When he was asked if he had any contact with Ebola patients he said 'yes' then he said 'no' then he would say 'yes' but refused to give out any names. The driver thinks the man is crazy."

Joseph started to laugh and then pointed at Josephine, saying, "Oh, they found you a husband!" Then he nearly split his sides laughing, continuing the joke until Josephine shot back something in Krio, prompting Joseph to say 'no' several times through his amusement. Josephine rolled her eyes then barked at Joseph to do his job and spray the rear of the ambulance so we could get the patient out for a look.

At Mary's suggestion, Joseph sprayed me down extra thoroughly in case we had to send the man back out. I would do the entire medical assessment in the rear of the ambulance and by good luck, he'd not be admitted and could return home to annoy his village. The lighting in the ambulance was fine and I approached the rear and instructed the 23 year old fellow that all I needed was his temperature and for him to answer a couple of questions. First, he would need to come back towards me and bend down so I could scan his temple. Joseph translated my instructions for good measure and the fellow tentatively came towards us and stood at the rear.

I put up the thermometer and placed the red light in the middle of his forehead but before I could press the button to start the process, he threw both hands up in front of his face, turned his head and ran back to the rear of the ambulance.

I pleaded with the fellow, reassuring him it was OK and that no one would hurt him. "It's OK. All I'm going to do is get your temperature. You'll be fine."

He returned to his previous spot at my urging to the rear of the ambulance. Again, I lifted the thermometer and placed the red dot on his temple and yet again he raised his hands to block the light, muting the attempt.

"Hey," I said, trying to sound authoritative, "the sooner you let me finish this sooner we might be able to let you go home. Be a swell fellow and help me out here, OK."

The man kept mumbling phrases that no one understood. I could discern enough that they were repetitive, redundant. Again I raised up my thermometer, put the dot to his head and again he blocked it with his hands and turned his head away.

"OK," I conceded, "we'll ask you a couple of questions first." I turned to Joseph and asked him to translate 'Do you have a fever? Do you have unexplained bleeding from the gums, nose or eyes? Do you have diarrhea? If so, is it bloody? Do you have general malaise or fatigue? Do you have an upset stomach?', and so on.

Joseph took each question in turn, nodding after each answer the man gave. The questioning started to take longer than I anticipated but I held my tongue and let Joseph continue to the end. After what seemed like too long, Joseph turned to me with the man's answers. "I don't know."

I was stymied. "You mean you don't know or he doesn't know?"

"Both." Joseph apparently expected me to make something out this.

I took my best stab at interpreting the results of our questions, openly surmising, "You mean he seems confused or unable to understand the questions. Am I close?"

Joseph looked at me and shrugged, his answer all doubt. "I guess. Maybe. He's very crazy."

The four of us were now all speechless but the patient certainly had plenty of spare words to fill in the silence, muttering as we all sat there like lumps on a log wondering what to do next.

I took an extra close look at the patient's wide open eyes—and yes they were what you'd call crazy eyes, that wide open look of someone startled or fearful, on alert. The good news was that the whites of his very open eyes was absent of any tinge of red. Additionally, there was no obvious fatigue or any other discharge. He was dry. All I needed was a temperature to come in at normal and I could send this patient home.

Yet again, I aimed the scanning thermometer to try to nail the patient's temp down and yet again he raised his hands to block the red beam. I decided that this was now a game of wits but first I tried to explain all the reasons why it was it to his benefit to let me complete my medical assessment.

Josephine started laughing, cackling out, "You are arguing with a crazy man!"

Mary interjected, "And you're losing."

I had no retort other than to concur that a person whose intellectual capacity was certainly questionable was sandbagging me. I decided no more pleading. I pressed the button on the thermometer as if I was going for the kill on a video game. One shot never does it but lob a couple hundred shots in the general direction and you might get lucky. We battled. I would point and shoot to scan and he would dodge and duck his head and thwart me with his open palms. This went on tens of times until I made the master move: I pointed the red dot at his feet, goading him into dropping his hands down to block the red dot on his toes. At that moment, I pulled out a second thermometer in my other hand and scanned his temple while he was focused on the red point on his foot. "Gothcha'!" I yelled out, raising my arms in victory.

I looked at the thermometer and sighed, telling everyone, "38.6 centigrade. Damn it! He has a fever."

The matter was settled. The temperature put him inside and since we had no reliable answers on whether or not he had recent contact in the past three weeks with other Ebola victims, we decided as a group that the temperature was the clinching fact for his admission.

Joseph and Josephine both now took a much more sympathetic tone and spoke to the poor fellow in his own language, urging him out of the ambulance and convincing him that the pills we wanted to give him were good for him and that the wristband was good luck, good magic.

A person didn't need to be native to the culture to recognize the patient was in the throes of psychosis, especially one that was marked by visibly defensive body language to routine medical exam. Without hesitation it was fair to say he was very paranoid beyond healthy and the repetitive phrases he muttered the entire time, along with his evasive answering of our questions, pigeon holed him as seriously mentally ill. Did the temperature mean he had Ebola? There's a thousand reasons a person can have a temperature but panic and hysteria over Ebola, and the reality of how widespread it had become in West Africa, coupled with how deadly and horrible death by Ebola was, erring on the side of patient autonomy and freedom was out the window. It was a quarantine medical model no one was arguing against.

Joseph and I each took an arm of the patient. We grasped his admission belongings in the other free hand, marching him up the concrete ramp and down to Suspect 4, a dry unit. He at first refused to go in and our thinking was that if we went in ahead and put down his personal belongings he would follow. After hesitating for several minutes, he stepped in and took his bed, keeping his eyes on us and never turning his back. Almost immediately the other patients, all male except for one female, picked up their belongings and headed out the door to find other places to sleep. It was surreal.

"What just happened here?" I asked Joseph.

"They know he's not right in the mind. They don't trust him," Joseph replied.

"He hardly said a word and he didn't even look at any of them when he walked in. What could they know in one minute?" I asked, genuinely perplexed.

"They heard what he said," Joseph answered.

"What was that?" I asked, incredulous that anything he said amounted to anything at all.

"That he would cast a spell on everyone in the room," Joseph informed.

"Seriously? They think he could do that to them?" I asked, even more incredulous.

"They aren't going to take any chances." Then Joseph thumped his chest with his palm and asked me to place my hand in the same spot where I could feel a hard lump of an object on a chain. He continued, "And I'm not taking any chances either. When we get out I'll show what I have and you should get one, too."

"I'll take my chances," I said, continuing, "Just in case, you show me what it is you use and I'll think about it."

Joseph tried bucking me up, saying, "You won't regret it."

The pressing problem was gathering up the bedside charts and tracking down the patients who left, then matching them back up with their notes, as well as making sure they were all in a dry unit. This took another half hour of our time and the two of us were moving slowly. It had to be late. Neither of us had any supper and no water. By my guess, it was at least 9:00 pm but there was no one at the gate waiting for admission. It was our one chance to get out so we headed for the doffing station. No one was waiting for us, meaning we had to yell out towards the sprayers' sleeping barracks to get some help doffing. Ten minutes rolled by before anyone stirred, giving me time to think over all the metal debris on the ground, especially the nails. One bad step and into the boot to my foot would mean an embarrassing million dollar plane ride home to quarantine in the states. If anyone else became infected, I could chalk that up to being on the bad side of high risk. Spend enough time doing this job, eventually the odds would catch a person off guard. It could be something as simple as one ever so small unfelt aerosolized virus-laden droplet up under the visor near the eye or some other stray inoculating dose of virus that somehow survived to get outside onto any object a person normally had contact with, be it a pen or sheet of paper or God only knows what. I just didn't want to be that person. No one did. Considering that we were surrounded and swimming in the Ebola virus, it was amazing we were as incident free as we were-- especially in light of how heavy the workload had become as the virus continued to bloom and reap more victims.

My legs shook as I stood and sloshed my boots in the chlorine tub. The first tell tale signs of cramps, a strange prodromal feeling of dread as tendons and muscle strained under some sort of invisible violence, a feeling I experienced enough of over the years from hard outdoor work and distance running one mile too many in high heat. All the sweat that left my body over the past 4 hours had more than likely carried gram upon gram of sodium and potassium outside of me, leaving the normal sodium-potassium ion exchange at the cellular level of my muscles a chaotic wreck that would respond with mega cramping.

The attitude and expectation that people in certain professions are invincible, immune to fatigue and the errors that percolate within, is promulgated the world over with stories of heroic endurance by policemen, soldiers, firemen, athletes and others I'm sure could be added to the aforementioned. In our respective work cultures, many of us are silently taught we should be able to ignore risks of personal damage that accompanies extreme fatigue, somehow magically never becoming mentally or physically numb. It is a belief rooted in an overinflated sense of physical being that many in such professions are more than happy to promote publicly and reinforce to one another privately. This attitude, never really formally taught, is infused into every student of medicine during their training, where schedules ignore the physical limits of physician interns. The 100 hour week, the utter nonsense that complicated skills can be learned and taught as 'See one, Do one, Teach one' and that multi tasking allows for separate agendas to have equally positive results doesn't stand up to even the lightest critiques.

Sadly, when reality meets legend, those attempting to manage a crisis with feats of super human strength find they are failures, overestimating themselves and neglecting the aid of those who secretly harbor the same self doubts, anxious to lend a hand to affirm the gnawing knowledge they, too, are merely human. All it takes to propagate this vicious cycle is one misplaced admonishment of another's work from some loud mouth who has way too high of an opinion of their own emotional, mental and physical strength. To make matters worse, too many of us are our own terrible enemies, internalizing unrealistic ideals, assigning guilt and blame where there should be none, and carrying weight which serves only to misdirect energies toward inventing more egregious standards. These standards end up ensconced in policy and law, enforced by self righteous prigs who hold themselves forth as saints and protectors, giving one another odd awards, throwing parades and back slapping themselves as heroes. It's all a harmful fiction that further forces an expectation that ignores literal physiological and spiritual boundaries, promulgating an us vs them world, one where certain professions cannot properly uphold standards within their own ranks that are precisely for the safety of those outside those ranks.

If anyone has a hard time comprehending the aforementioned, let me summarize with a real world example that affects our lives on a daily basis: Zero tolerance. Zero tolerance is an idea that belongs in the realm of terror fiction as a literary device. Zero tolerance means zero lack of judgment with zero basis in reality. Zero tolerance equals zero brains. Man, the unerring machine, becomes an ideological comic book.

Now here I was in the nurse's station, afraid that one more ambulance would arrive and I would have to cajole Joseph go back in with me. He was indeed tough, or he was putting on one heck of a show that he was unaffected by the last 4 hours. I dug into the freezer for cold bottled water and mixed up 3 liters of electrolyte solution for the two of us and threw in some cherry flavoring. We then both chugged away and finished off the bottles. Then lightening hit me.

My hands cramped so hard I could not make a fist and when I finally managed to force movement in one finger, the muscles of my forearm turned into bands of inflexible steel wrapping themselves into a vice so tight that it felt like my forearm was being crushed. The other arm followed almost immediately. I kicked a spot clean on the floor and got on to a spare blanket to lie down, hoping I could stretch my muscles enough to stave off the involuntary contractions. It failed. My feet cramped. My calves cramped. The hamstrings and quads followed. Then something that never happened to me or anyone I ever knew or even heard of, my face and lips cramped. I was now one huge groaning mess, unable to sit up and only able to roll side to side. This went on for 20 more minutes until Joseph came back. There was genuine concern and even a little fear in his face at how he found me.

"I'm going to get you some help," Joseph said, turning back toward the door.

"No!" I shouted at him. "What I need is salt. Find me some raw salt. I think that'll do the job. Please hurry. This really sucks, man."

Joseph ran next door to the meal tent and I could hear him rummaging about. Soon he was back with a table salt shaker, one of those throw away kind. Holding out his cupped hand, he poured until his hand was nearly full. I opened my mouth and he dribbled it on my tongue and gums. Then he put a bottle of water to my lips and I took enough to moisten the salt, hoping this would allow the mucous tissues of my mouth to take it up faster. We repeated this cycle two more times and used up the entire shaker which was about 1/3 full at the start.

Within a few minutes I could feel the pipe wrenches and vice grips unclamping. I started by testing my hands by flexing them. Residual tension was present but they stopped spasming enough that I could open and close them. I could smile and shape my lips into a whistle with no tightening. The final test was flexing my biceps and extending and flexing my legs. I had control of my voluntary motor functions again, enough for Joseph to help me get back into a chair and sit in front of a fan to dry. With the fan oscillating, the two of us worked on our second bottles of electrolyte solution as we washed in its breeze.

"Are you hungry?" I asked Joseph.

"I live in Sierra Leone," Joseph offered. "We always say we are hungry."

"Why would you do that?" I asked, curious.

"Because everyone is hungry enough of the time that when someone asks if we're hungry, it means they probably have food to offer. You never turn down food even if you are full because eventually you will be hungry again."

"You mean you take it anytime you can get it," I summed up.

"Don't you do that in America?" he asked, toying the pendant on his chest.

I chuckled. "No. In America if you ask someone if they're hungry, they tell you they're on a diet. Americans like to pass time eating and talking about their latest diet. The other answer you're as likely to get if you ask if someone is hungry is 'No, I just ate and I'm trying to lose 10 pounds for my class reunion.'"

Joseph gave me a quizzical look, then asked, "Does everybody in America spend their free time eating and getting so fat they need to stop eating?"

Shaking my head to show it was a mystery to me as much as him, I replied, "Yeah, that's about it."

Then we returned to silence for a few minutes until Joseph asked me if I was better. I nodded that I was and thanked him for helping me out.

"Your pendant. That thing around your neck," I questioned, pointing to the lump under his soaked gray t-shirt, "You said inside that it protected you."

Shaking his head for emphasis in the affirmative, Joseph claimed, saying, "There is evil in the world and people who practice it. That crazy man is trapped in a spell and might not be safe.

This protects me."

"Can I see it?"

Joseph reached into his shirt and pulled up the silver chain until the pendant came out then displayed it for me to see.

I looked and recognized it immediately. "That's St. Jude. Patron saint of lost causes."

With a mix of surprise and admiration, Joseph asked, "You know who this is?"

"Oh, yes," I bragged, continuing, "I was raised Catholic. Know all about St Jude. My family had little statutes and medals of St. Jude, sort of like yours, and we'd pray over them when things weren't going so well."

"I am Catholic, too," Joseph exclaimed, happy to share a commonality between the two of us. "Do you still have your St Jude medals?"

I shook my head, "No. The last time I prayed to him I was out driving and got lost. I prayed to St. Jude to help me find the place I was looking for. Never found it, so I punished him by locking him in the glove box."

Joseph laughed at the story and we continued with small talk, mostly him telling me how far he had gone in school. He had some college and wanted more so he could be a businessman and that he had 7 people in his family, all alive, but that he was the only one with a job and that he got the Maforki job through a family connection with Dr. George. His big dream was to leave Africa and go to Great Britain to work as an executive. But for now, he had to use all his earnings to help out the family, meaning college was not in the near future.

Then the nurses' station cell phone rang, the caller ID displaying 'Admissions'. I picked up and listened to Mary give me the run down then hung up the phone.

"Another ambulance?" Joseph asked, concerned.

"No. It was good news. The ambulance that was supposed to come here never left the last village. No more ambulances tonight," I smiled, ready to do a cartwheel or two to celebrate. "We can go home."

The two of us walked back to the admissions building and past the police guards who were bundled up against the cool weather. A chill persisted due to my moist clothes but I forced myself to tolerate it, knowing that heat would soon enough return to make me wish it was cooler. Ibrahim was in his van, heater running full blast, and Mary and I stepped in to head home.

"Hello, Reeck," Ibrahim drawled out.

"Hi," I said, "Glad to see you. I'm getting pretty hungry."

Ibrahim shook his head, knowing he was disappointing me, and said, "No extra food. Not much was on the table. No extras. Victor and I had to share a plate. Sorry."

Mary commiserated, saying, "I'd go and get you something from the Dutch kitchen but they lock after 9 o'clock. I'm down to a couple of granola bars myself."

Back at the compound, I found a stray jar of peanut butter and a violated pack of crackers. About a ¼ jar of peanut butter remained. With larger portions of cracker, I scraped out what I could then used a finger, alternating a finger of peanut butter with a few crumbs of cracker. Sated enough to go to bed, having no water buckets at the ready, I wiped down with alcohol pads and rolled into my sheet.
∎∎

Red Jacket

I woke up but everyone was already gone, not hearing them when they had breakfasted. My entire body felt pretty much like the day after you run a marathon, each muscle telling me to stay off my feet, to take my time. I had all day to rest until I went in later in the afternoon, the last of evening shifts before shifting back to days. Outside my door, someone left a note reminding me that there was a weekly meeting that day. Basically, the meetings were information catch ups on how well supplies were being managed, new people coming in, progress report on getting the contact teams up and running. Little was said about the nuts and bolts of running the place, probably because somehow we managed to organize a system that worked well enough with what was available.

Meetings were less must-do since the British contribution to establishing wireless internet at Maforki ETU and compounds facilitated greater ease of communication, lessening the need for meetings to disseminate information. However, the day the British came to our compound to set up the antenna for the wireless, they found out within the hour that there was too much geographical interference to receive a worthwhile signal, forcing us to continue with our wireless hotspots that worked off of cell towers and were generally unpredictable because you never knew who else would go online and decide they just had to see some video, hogging up the bandwidth. Again, our poor compound had yet another black mark against it.

The house workers were busy at the pump filling everyone's buckets, doing laundry and other household chores. I wordlessly walked outdoors to the patio deck to pick over the breakfast. Nothing. Everything was already cleaned up and put away. I asked Victor if there were any leftovers but the house help had eaten the last of it themselves.

"Not even an egg or some plantains?" I asked, hoping for something.

"No. Nothing," Victor commiserated. "The lockdown disrupted everything but it should get better tomorrow. There is still hot water if you would like some tea."

I shrugged and Victor pointed out the kettle on the table. We sat and sipped instant coffee while looking for a hotspot but there were none out on the table, nixing any idea of trying to read email or cruise the news. Geckos scurried up and down the walls, curious enough to stop in their tracks for a few moments to eyeball us then scamper off to wherever it is geckos need to go.

With little else to do, I decided to take a walk down to the market, hoping to score something to eat but the New Years Day lockdown still had the markets closed. Some scattered merchants were trying to do business but being circumspect about it, not trying to stand out to the police. The fried dough lady was who I was looking for but no fires were going along the road that indicated anything scone-like was being cooked up. So back I went to my room to read my Neil Armstrong biography and piddle around until lunch, hoping something would show up for me to eat.

Lunch hour arrived but no lunch. This wasn't going to work. I needed to eat. Off to the club I hiked only to find the doors closed. The two fellows at the door told me I could come in for drinks but because of the lockdown, they wouldn't be serving food until tomorrow when the 3 day lockdown officially ended. I left with two cans of lukewarm cola and decided to go back to my room and get into my scrubs and head down to the ETU, hopefully to score some lunch. Time was getting tight if I was to make it.

I called for a driver, hoping to hasten my getting to the ETU for lunch. By the time Ibrahim was able to get to me, it would have been faster for me to walk the half hour. Ibrahim dropped me off and I hurried my way through temp check, ignoring greetings as best I could to make the lunch tent before it shut down. I rapped on the window frame and was greeted by the drill sergeant of a lunch lady. Apparently, the world over, lunch ladies are screened by body type and personality traits and ours was no exception. She arms as big as telephone poles and a permanent frown that let you know just exactly how disappointed she was in you.

"You have any lunches left?" I asked, my timidity rivaling some 19th century Dickensian waif begging on a London street corner.

She stared me down and after I wilted a bit further she decided to answer, saying, "It's 2 o'clock. Lunch is over for an hour." She then slammed her window cover shut, leaving me to go into the nurses' station to scrounge the freezer for flavored water of which there was plenty enough.

Our meeting filled up the room but there were enough chairs so no one had to stand. Previously, prior to ETU staff being plucked for duties opening up new ETU's out in the countryside, there were so many of us that it was a coin flip to get a chair. Admissions up. ETU staff down.

The central topic of the meeting was days off and the expansion of the schedule to include a graveyard shift. I bit my tongue, wondering how they conducted the math of less Maforki ETU staff with more hours and mandatory days off. In the past week, I was tasked with putting a schedule together and finding everyone a day off, ideally once a week. It took only a matter of minutes for me to conclude there simply weren't enough of us to fill a day and evening shift with one day a week off, forcing me to schedule days off at about one every 12 days.

Next, a form was passed that covered basic conduct. One of the items was we had to agree to take one day off every week. No exceptions. Only in the last 5 days or so did some people get some days off. I prioritized by who had served the longest thus far and if they had a pressing need to some other obligation, such as meeting with other health system contacts or renewing some old friendships related to past West Africa work they would never have the chance to rekindle otherwise. The hard reality was there were simply not enough of us to put a day a week off system into place.

I stared at the form and the line about the days off. In my mind, my thinking was that if I signed it I would essentially be agreeing that there was one day off a week for everyone. The majority of us had worked every single day since our arrival and I'm fairly certain that the landing party who arrived two weeks before us did their whole tour, recently completed in the past several days, with maybe one day off. Two days tops. No, it wasn't a good idea to sign something that I felt put the workers in the position of demanding their day off in the midst of a labor shortage.

My concern over the scheduling ended when our director decided to take on the scheduling task. I was left with the impression that somehow he felt he could do a better job and in one way he had a tool I did not—he was the director and his word was pretty much the last. When the new schedule came out the following day, I spotted the trick immediately. By taking each of us and working our day shift into an evening shift the following day or two and then to the expanded night shift for a day or two, each move to a later shift gave us an extra eight hours before having to show up for work. Technically, by getting off at 8 am from the last scheduled night shift then starting back on days at 8 am the following day, a person had a full 24 hours off. Problem is, by the time you finish the last of your night shift at 8 in the morning, you go to bed and sleep to around supper time, waking up to eat and socialize a bit after sleeping the day away. The next day the cycle of day-evening-night resumed. That was no day off. The gimmick was spotted and for those who hadn't yet arrived to their day off on the calendar per the old schedule, they lost that day off and morale took a bit of hit.

Fact of the matter was people were getting tired. The surge in cases was testing everyone, eating away at our downtime between rounds in the hot zone as we tried to keep up with pharmaceutical prep and putting together patient material needs of fresh clothes, nutrition, bedding, etc. Being timely was becoming a challenge but it was doable as long as we worked together and kept an eye out for potential problems that could throw a wrench into the day. Procrastination was not a strategy.

The meeting ended with the relief that the scheduling was out of my hands. I handed my form back, signed but with the item crossed out about the day per week off inked out and initialed, hoping that if anyone actually looked it would give them pause enough to learn that the current situation regards such was essentially nothing more than a nice idea.

I was hungry and fatigued. It was my looking forward to going in that kept me enthusiastic. I liked it inside, seeing who had taken a turn for the worse or the better. Someone I had almost completely forgotten popped into mind—the Kargbo clan.

Over at the admissions' building I went down the board, scratching out my notes, still not knowing who I would be collaborating with for the evening shift. The entire Kargbo family was still holed up in Confirmed 3 and all still alive. The odds of their intact survival alone were inspiring. I finished my notes and checked in with Gwyn to see how the day had unfolded and what to expect going forward. The good news was that my partner and I for the evening would be free of having to handle the ambulances coming in and that two national nurses would handle anyone dropped off, though no communication had been made that any patients would be arriving from outlying areas after 5 o'clock or so. Judging by the 25 or so names on the day's admission board, most anyone who needed to be admitted had been. We topped out at about 70 patients. Happy New Year.

I returned to the supply building and gathered up my best guestimate of meds needed for inside rounds, filling two of the red biohazard bags with antibiotics, antimalarials, anxiolytics and antipyretics. For equal reasons a treat and a prophylactic action, I bought two cans of cola, trying to fend off any possible repeat of the cramping I had the night before. Maybe tonight I would be able to get a meal, have a normal supper.

Back at the nurses' station I stumbled over the concrete forms and stacks of lumber being used for the addition. I dug through a pile of boots until I identified mine by the infinity sign painted on with finger nail polish, shaking them out to make sure there were no scorpions inside to surprise me.

The nurses' station was quiet, a couple of folks I didn't know hunched over their laptops likely putting together numbers for the daily DERC report and sent out to the world. It was a good time to go over my meds and get all the premixing done so my partner and I could hit the ground running inside the ETU.

Not knowing who my partner would be was a problem. I checked the schedule again and only found initials, unable to place them with anyone I knew or had met. The whiteboard outside the nurses' station revealed even less. I went back in and gently interrupted the two men on their laptops, asking if by chance they knew anything about who was assigned for the evening round. One shook his head no and went back to his screen. The other stopped, stared at me for a moment then smiled, introducing himself, "I'm Dr. Ngyen. You're Rick?"

"Yeah. Nice to meet you. How do you fit into all this?" I asked.

"Infectious disease specialist. A group of us came in two nights ago and are staying at the Dutch camp. You're one of the nurses?"

"Yes," I replied, impressed that a real live infectious disease specialist was going to be part of my round. We exchanged our backgrounds and I found out he worked as a physician researcher in a large Midwest university hospital, specializing in the details of infectious tropical disease, which Ebola was on his study radar for the past couple of years. Calling the current crisis an opportunity of a lifetime for him would be somewhat ghoulish, but that was exactly what it was.

"You can call me Q," the doctor offered, putting a smile on and his hand out.

"OK. Good," I said, following up with, "Have you been inside yet? Anyone take you on an orientation run?"

"Yesterday we went on a dry run and they watched us don and doff, talked us through to make sure we were OK with all the gear. I think it went well," Q asserted, offering an optimistic assessment.

This was a little unsettling, throwing a new person into the mix who hadn't yet made a live round. I didn't mind precepting someone and, in fact, usually liked acclimating new nurses to the hospital floor. Q wasn't a nurse and this wasn't a hospital floor like back in the States. But it was what it was.

I grabbed my two red bags of meds and explained how we generally made a best guess of what would be needed, that any extra would be left in the med boxes as inventory, and that it was always a good idea to take in some extra oral antibiotics, Paracetamol, IV fluids and oral Valium to leave behind. I then showed him the Artemisinin and Rocephin we would pre mix and preload at the nurses' station to save time and avoid handling a needle one less time while in the hot zone.

Q stopped me, asking with not a little incredulity, "You do this not knowing who is going to need what exactly?"

I shook my head, saying, "Yes. We have 70 people inside that you and I have to touch base with. We'll know what they need by reading the medication administration record on their bedside charts."

Shaking his head in disbelief, Q asked, "Let me get this right—we don't know what the patient needs before we go in?"

"Not entirely true," I explained, hoping to alleviate Q's concern. "Over at the admissions' building, I take down a list of names of patients I'll be seeing and pay attention to when they were admitted and who has positive PCR results for Ebola and malaria. I check the positive malarias against the day they were admitted to come up with Artemisinin needed. As for antibiotics, nearly all the patients are getting them in one form or another, the difference being who can take them PO and those who need IM's or IV's."

Q was caught off guard by all this, eliciting a reaction that was perfectly normal but also perfectly wrong. "I think we can be a little more meticulous and organized than that. Let's go back to the admissions building and go over all the names again so we know exactly how much Artemisinin we're going to need."

He was the doctor. I was the nurse. But it was important to keep us on time so that the national nurse and sprayers with us weren't thrown off schedule. Everyone wanted to complete the first evening round in time for supper, especially myself since I was on my third day of not having a real meal. "We have to start getting prepared. I have everything we're going to need. Our best bet is to get inside and let the bedside charts direct us as to what needs to be done. Trust me on this if nothing else. Trying to figure out who needs exactly what when is next to impossible since we haven't been able to reliably pass information out of the hot zone to this side of the fence. We've tried whiteboards, taping notes to the fence and copying them once we're out, plain old memorization but all of it comes up short. The bedside charts and a robust inventory inside are the best options."

Q wasn't buying it. "Well, let's go look at the admissions board anyways." Without waiting for a rebuttal from me, he got up and left, taking the lead for me to follow. Over at the admissions building, we went over my notes and he compiled his own version then sat down to try to figure out exactly what medications were needed for each patient.

After an hour, I couldn't handle it anymore, impatiently prodding, "Q, we really need to get inside so we can get staff back out for supper. You have to believe me that this type of forecasting is more mental gymnastics than practical."

Q looked up from his notes, saying, "Just a couple of more and I'll be ready."

Another few minutes ticked off when a national nurse, one I didn't recognize, barged into the room and not smiling, half demanding half shouting, "You Rick?"

I nodded that I was.

She repeatedly slapped her bare wrist as if she were noting the time. "We need to go. Now."

Q was oblivious. I asked her if she was part of the evening rounds team and she said she was.

Then I made a promise I couldn't keep, saying, "Go ahead and get donned. Tell the sprayer, too, that we're on our way over now."

Hoping to push Q a bit, I stood up and announced that I'd be waiting for him at the donning tent and he replied that he'd be there, not saying when, then put his head back down to his note taking.

Being behind and hoping to catch up, I sprinted back over to the nurses' station, yelling 'hello' to J Edgar and everyone else shouting out. Ali was

and 4, I started immediately assessing the inventory situation to locate likely needed supplies.

I grabbed the first bedside chart and saw the name 'Kargbo' and noticed the first name 'Sally'. When I looked up from the paperwork to put face and paper together, no Sally. I grabbed the next chart and saw 'Kargbo, Josephine'. No Josephine. Then I grabbed the whole lot of charts for that area and went through her children's' names. None was present. The last chart finally did have a person attached to it, the uncle of the kids, sitting upright on his mattress, holding his mostly empty water bottle, alert and responsive, even refreshed looking. I was startled enough by his healthy posture and affect that I checked the name on his wrist band against the chart to verify that this was the one and same brother of Josephine. The half dollar sized spot of graying hair in the middle top of his head was further proof I was thinking of the right person. Then I looked right and then I looked left, scanning for Josephine and the kids. Fearing the worst, I rechecked their charts to see the last time anyone recorded any sort of activity on them.

I studied each column, checking to ascertain the last date of any entry wasn't several days ago, meaning the patient was discharged by foot or by bag and that the chart wasn't taken down, a problem every once in awhile that left us wondering if someone was discharged to home, passed away or was lost in the shuffle of things. All the Kargbos had an entry from today recorded on day shift.

This was near miraculous. The odds of all six recovering were long even though the mortality rate had dropped from 90% two months earlier to a generous 30% in the last 10 days or so. The family was not included as my set of patients, that just being the luck of draw partially, but I was in C-3 enough to breeze by them on my way to others. Each time I paid attention, they looked worse than the last and figured it was only a matter of a couple of days that family would be missing one or two. Even the chatter at the supper table supported the idea, maybe bracing all of us for the worst, that mom, uncle or at least a child would succumb.

I asked the uncle how he was feeling, him understanding my question well enough that he smiled and nodded in the affirmative. I put my hand down to take his and to encourage him, he grasping that I wanted him to stand. With only a modest amount of assistance from me, he was able to get his legs underneath him and stand up off the mattress, steady and straight, needing no help from me to do so. By this meager assessment, I guessed he was well enough to have another PCR drawn to ascertain if his viral load was low enough so he could go home. He sat back down, reached for his Styrofoam container and began feeding himself.

This excited me enough that I went outside to find Josephine. She wasn't out front. I dipped in between the buildings to the rear and quickly spotted a woman in a bright red coat, gold and white dress with a head wrap to match. Even on the outside where Sierra Leonean women paid attention to their dress and presentation, it was an impressive piece of wardrobe, as if she were adorned in royal attire. She was laughing at someone or something and as I cleared the rear of the buildings, I could hear, then see, her three kids punching one of the soccer balls around that Francie had brought in weeks earlier. Each of them was clean and in clothes that on the outside would be eye catching.

I approached Josephine, doubting she would know who I was and I was correct. I made an introduction and did everything I could with my voice and animated gestures to show her how happy I was at being able to see her in such good condition. She smiled and laughed, saying, "We are all blessed today," and clapped her hands.

Then I noticed there was no Sally. "Where's Sally?"

Josephine smiled and then pointed towards the showers half absent-mindedly. When I looked, the reason why she pointed less than enthusiastically was that from our vantage point we could see Sally at the faucet washing up. Even from the distance we were, it was easy to see Sally was in fine shape, her young skin unblemished and eyes clear.

I turned back to Josephine and asked, pointing at the crook of my elbow, "Have they taken your blood again yet?"

Josephine rolled up her sleeve, revealing the tell tale piece of gauze taped to where they took her blood sample.

"Wonderful," I emphasized. "The kids? Sally? Uncle?"

Josephine set her near black eyes on me, speaking with a contentment hinting optimism, saying, "All are done. Only Uncle is left."

"They haven't drawn uncle's blood yet," I interpreted, adding, "I'll make a note of it that he gets one tonight."

Seeing I wasn't understanding, Josephine lowered her voice, serious, saying, "Oh, no, they took his blood but his wasn't good yet."

Again, I interpreted this to mean the sample somehow was screwed up and a result wasn't feasible. "Sometimes there isn't enough blood for a decent test so they have to draw again. They'll get it the next time."

Josephine shook her head, indicating that I needed enlightenment. "No, the doctor said today he still has a very small piece of the disease left but that in one day, tomorrow, his blood should be well enough to go home."

Then the proverbial light bulb went off in my head. "You have results?" I tentatively asked, fearing that this all was some sort of weird remission that could still come up short.

"Oh, yes. Everyone is cured. Except Uncle. He is just mostly cured." She patted her chest near her heart, showing her gratitude for the path of events.

My surprise was obvious even through all the gear. Josephine stamped her foot to the ground and made me aware of her resolve and her declaration, practically ordering, "We will not leave one at a time or two at a time. Everybody in this family will stay until the very end and go back to home the same way we came in—as one family."

If anyone had any doubts about who was in charge of the Kargbo clutch, there was none left that it was Josephine. She was dressed for triumph and saw to it that everyone else would be too, her optimism self-fulfilling thanks to her metal rod of a spine.

I congratulated her again and returned to C-3 to review notes I brought inside, along with the family's charts. Sure enough, 5 of the 6 were PCR(-), meaning they could have gone home today. Only the uncle was PCR(+). I learned that Josephine objected to leaving Uncle behind, insisting that all six were to walk through the gate as one family.

Inside, Uncle was sprawled out and covered meaningfully by a light lafa, quietly napping and his supper closed back up. I leaned over him and lifted the container, quietly testing its weight, checking how much he had eaten. All of it. His water bottle was empty. Then in a narrative note in his chart I read the Major's note stating how Josephine had taken it on herself to learn how to change bags of IV fluids and give proper doses of Paracetamol for everyone. Josephine taught Sally. Between the two of them, they'd doctored and nursed the remaining family, stretching themselves into what for a patient is unfamiliar territory. This was intentional since the Major, Jim and Keri made the family their pet project, most likely out of trepidation that the loss of even one from such a tight knit group would be devastating to the whole family's morale. Probably, equally so, our own morale, even though it certainly was no fluke that other families who came in together too many times went home several members short of what arrived.

As I digested this information of a patient taking care of other patients and that a medical person taught them how to do so, I understood why it wasn't exactly common knowledge. Under the circumstances, it might have been a good idea to expand the concept, especially within families that were here together. I put the charts down with admiration for the whole of it all and those who were part of it. As far as I was concerned, this was rock star stuff that belonged on a poster like the one with Led Zeppelin posing in front of their private 747.

Yet again, I was treading down the road of being inside too long. Isha plowed through her list of patients, bags of normal saline hung plump and full, and the red biohazard bag she took charge of was empty. I looked down the walkway to the doffing station and Albert was prepping her for her exit, chlorine spray being generously applied from the shoulders down. It was starting to get dusky, the sun still a sliver over the horizon. Supper was being served. I could smell the brown rice and vegetables with baked chicken.

Hunger was taking over my thinking. You know this when you began thinking of ways to feed yourself from untouched patient meals left to spoil inside the ETU. The rational part of me quickly nixed any ideas of even attempting such a ludicrous move. What was troubling was that I even had it as an idea at all. Eating food inside an Ebola ward as a possible option? That falls only in spot one on any sort of continuum—odd to sick. Under these circumstances, I was considering ORS fortified cola to be a health food.

The list of patients in Q's and mine biohazard bag had some noted additions from Q regards their current status. I shrugged this off as a habit from his medical training, something we all experienced and he would soon disabuse himself of, learning that trying to keep accurate, up to date notes on the outside was difficult at best since things like taping scribbled, chlorine-soaked notes to the fence just blew away, crinkled and balled up by the slightest breeze. The entire bedside chart initiative was meant to, and did, save us from this inaccurate and incomplete redundancy of rerecording information that was of very little, if any use, on the outside. No one could write orders based off such information or put together long term treatment plans. In fact, the treatment plan at the basic was universal: more fluids, secondary infection control, nutrition and as much emotional support as could be mustered to bridge the cultural gaps and the white, anonymous armor of the staff. In too many cases, the alternative treatment plan was merely comfort measures. No point in a Plan of Treatment document for the terminally ill when adequate painkillers were absent and other devices, such as suctioning equipment to clear throats or supplemental oxygen to ease breathing, were nowhere to be found. What was best was to react to what you suspected or understood about a patient's condition and go at it with what you had on hand the moment you were delivering care. The analogy that could be made about Maforki resources is that back home, the tools available literally needed entire campuses of buildings to house. However, here we could put all the needed tools in a medium sized plastic trash can bag.

I looked around and couldn't see Q so I decided I had better find him. He wasn't far, just next door in C-4, but he was hunched over a pile of charts, studiously copying away. Our red bag of meds was still on the heavy side. The first reaction was to find a patient with their chart at the bed and take care of them, but my walk around showed there were no charts on any of the patient's beds to guide me. Q had them all.

"Hey, Q," I interrupted. "Can I get a couple of the charts and get going on some of the folks here?"

Without Q looking up, all I heard was, "Almost done." It was a phrase we would all hear many times. To kill time, I tidied up the med box table and then helped a mother try to get some formula into her toddler, a modest success once Mom was able to hold the child's head still enough for me to bleed some formula out of a syringe and past the child's ominously bluish lips. The mother herself was visibly uncomfortable, each breath a conscious effort. I put another bag of IV fluids up for her and she lay back down on her side, pulling the child in close to her bosom only to have it throw up all the formula it just ingested. Some unused rags were nearby and the two of us cleaned up the silent child first then worked on drying off mom's damp blouse. It was all a very quiet effort, even mechanical, with no sense of optimism or gratitude left upon which to draw. I covered her with a blanket and arranged her bag so she could use it as a pillow and maybe fashion a temporary escape with some sleep.

Q finally moved on. He was getting little in the way of information from the elderly patient due to the patient's lack of English skills and his lack of Krio skills, forcing him to rely on the bedside chart notes the national nurses translated on a previous visit. Q turned to me, asking, "Can we get one of the national nurses back in here so I can talk to this gentleman?"

I shook my head 'no', and then followed with, "Part of our job is to take advantage of that when they're in here with us. They're more than happy to help out. I'd even say it's a point of pride for them."

I could see the wheels turning in Q's head. After several moments, he shared his brainstorm, saying, "Let's have them split the round with us. One comes in for the first half of our round and the second comes in for the second half."

"Are you suggesting that you plan on staying in here so long that we need to tag team national nurses?" I asked, hoping I was misunderstanding him.

"Well, yeah. It looks like we need to stay in an extra hour to finish everyone," Q observed, waving his hands as if to demonstrate how large a task it had all become.

I chuckled a bit. "You better hope your enthusiasm is as infectious as this outbreak. After two hours of sweating, everyone is ready to get out and take a recuperation break. The cooler, dry weather of today is an anomaly that'll be gone tomorrow. Even then, two hours becomes an outer limit. Pace matters. I already paid the price once for challenging the obvious." I waxed on, regaling Q with the previous night's adventure of what happens to a person after 5 hours non-stop wrapped in pieces of plastic, rubber and cotton. I could tell he wasn't grasping the physicality of it all quite yet.

Dusk was heavy and the first stars of the night were visible. Supper wasn't going to happen. By the time we would finish the first round it would be time to go back in on the second, undermining my already tentative mood. This was utter nonsense, a debacle I allowed by not insisting on adherence to completing the Plan of Treatment detailed in the bedside charts, prioritizing fluids and comfort measures. Second-guessing what should be done for each patient has its place when there is the luxury of times and resources. We were short on both. The only place left was outside at the nurses' station, or around the evening supper table, to reconsider the best medical approach to the patients. Even then, individually tailored treatment plans were rare, with treatment plans considered in categories such as mothers and infants, children or the elderly and at what stage of the disease they were in. All of it was one state of constant triage, evaluating and revaluating as we visited each patient based on the broad outlines we learned in the first few days. This was as far away as imaginable from the trend of boutique medicine back in the states where, if a patient could afford it, specialized attention could be sold more akin to the service the elite may find at five star hotels.

We reached and covered our last patient, having spent twice as long as Isha did on her assignment. At the doffing station, moths battered themselves against the yellow lights. The quiet of the camp revealed that many of the workers had taken to their beds. No sprayers were present to walk us through doffing, forcing me to yell out through the fence until someone came down the walkway and geared up to put us through the decontamination process. The sprayer's orders and direction were terse, devoid of the usual back and forth banter, hinting that he was less than happy to be thrown off his rest schedule. When the point of doffing came where Q and I had to stand on one foot each as the bottoms of our boots were sprayed, I noticed the sprayer was definitely dragging it out, forcing us to hop from one leg to the next to keep upright. All this was in silence.

The cool night air set a chill into the wet clothes pasted to my skin, putting me into a suit of gooseflesh. Rather than waiting for my rounds partner as I normally would, I set stride down to the mess tent hoping to score a stray plate. Inside the light was off but it didn't take cat eye vision to see the tables were empty. A quick jab of white from the bottom of one of the tarp walls flashed a moment of light as a feral dog pushed his way out, thinking better of it that we share the room.

From inside the ETU a brief flurry of snaps and growls between the dogs put us on notice they were getting ready to work the hot zone for any leftovers. I had become so inured of their presence that I couldn't recall if they were present during our last round.

My thought of the dogs was interrupted by a blue reflection of strobing ambulance light off the light poles that stretched over the top of the buildings. Any second, I was expecting our phone to ring and be ordered to the admissions' building to tend an arrival. Soon I could hear the Krio chatter of national nurses, relieved someone had stepped in to do the job and allow Q and me some time to recharge.

Q followed up behind me and took a chair from the desk, immediately taking out his own notebook to jot down what he could recall. After a few minutes, he began to ask me about such and such patient over in this or that corner wearing a blue sweat jacket or some other completely unmemorable color or pattern of clothing. I almost half expected him to fall back on race as an identifying characteristic except that Q was smarter than that.

Up on the wall, a moth with long, pink fronds dipped in pollen-colored yellow clung to the bottom of the clock. It was nearly 9 o'clock, our late start and overly long 1st round overlapped our 2nd round, cutting out rest and dry time. I hadn't even taken off my boots, then realized there was no point since it was time to head back through to tie up the loose ends. Over in the donning tent, I could hear Isha and the sprayer talking. Normally, she would have tracked us down to let us know she was ready but she knew better, figuring that by sticking to her own plan she would be more efficient without Q and me to stumble over. Our most valuable asset, a translator and cultural guide, was sending a clear message that procrastination was unacceptable.

Then I did it. "Q, I'll be back."

Q, head in his notes, half whispered, "OK."

I jumped on over to the donning tent where Isha and the sprayer were ready to pull down their visors and forge the gate.

"I'll be quick," I said. I ripped into a package for a suit, snapped it in the air to its full length and dashed one leg at a time through the ankle cuffs, then zipped myself in full. Isha joined me and peeled off an apron, spreading it out so I could pop my head through. As she was tying me off, the sprayer wrote my name on the apron while I put the last of two pairs of gloves on. My hood and the N-95 mask followed and Isha handed me a visor. A quick look inside her red biohazard bags showed an inventory that was more than adequate. On this round, there would be no shots to give, that task finished up during the previous.

"Split them like before?" I suggested.

"Yes," she said, her tone implying, 'Why would you even ask that?' Then she addressed the elephant in the room, or the lack of the subject in the room, asking, "Is the other man ready or are you just not going to wait?" The tone of her voice was more tentative, suspicious that at the last moment I would demand she go nowhere until Q arrived.

"If any of us wants to finish this next round before sunrise," I mockingly advised, "we'll go in right now."

I could see Isha's cheeks rise on the outside of her mask, indicating a smile. She shoved a 'thumbs up' in my face and off we went, our pace determined and deliberate. We split the patients up, going bed to bed on our respective charges and administered the needed medications, cleaning them as we went along where they needed it, replacing bags of IV fluids and dosing liberally with diazepam, metoclopromide and Paracetamol in hopes they could have a night of sleep free of pain and nausea.

At the Kargbo bedsides, Josephine sensed Isha was not interested in any idleness, thus holding her lips other than to smile and nod a 'thank you'. Soon enough Isha and I were at the doffing station and, along with our sprayer, all of our moods lightened to have finished the job a half an hour before I had to leave. The three of us walked down the breezeway and peeled off to our own tents, me being the furthest down.

Inside the nurses' station, I peeked in half expecting Q to berate me for leaving him behind. But he wasn't there and I didn't care. I dumped my bag and took out dry scrubs and headed to the showers, enduring the chill but thrilled to cut the grime of the day away for a feeling of dry, warm fresh clothes.

Dressed and refreshed I head over to the admissions building. Inside Q was in a fleece pull over, poring over the patient roster up on the whiteboards, jotting down notes in the same notebook he had back over in the nurses' station. He looked up at me, asking, "Are you ready?"

"To go home? Yeah."

"No," he corrected. "I think there are some things we can do if we go back in quick."

"Are you aware I just finished a second round with Isha?", challenging Q to defend his sense of schedule.

"I didn't know you left for that," Q claimed, looking bewildered.

For Q, I concluded a sense of time was not an instinctive attribute. Just as I was getting ready to chide him how timeliness is the courtesy of kings, Ibrahim barged in, the light of the room unmasking the sleep in his eyes. Half-shouting, Ibrahim pointed to the van outside, "Time to go. Right now." With that he turned back out the door and slammed his driver's side door.

Q wanted to object. You could see he had 'just one more thing to do'. I jumped him.

"Q. Now. The driver's waiting. Tomorrow you can work on your ideas," I said, knowing that his procrastination and over thinking would be some other poor person's job killer. "He'll leave us here, so come on."

Ibrahim got Q back to the Dutch camp then him and me back to our shared compound, the two of us talking about the price of American visas for someone from Sierra Leone and other ways someone from

Sierra Leone might make it into the United States to work or study. It was Ibrahim's favorite subject.

I think everyone in our group admired Ibrahim for his sense of fairness and approachability. Those he worked with to make our stay workable and comfortable appeared to respect him. His mother was a chief and Ibrahim seemed to have the temperament to be a natural fit to follow her when the time came. When I asked if he wanted such a position, he protested that he did not feel he had the skills or patience.

One morning, as a half dozen of us were walking to work, a man was chasing a boy of about 10. The boy was desperate in his attempts to elude his pursuer who was single mindedly determined to capture the boy. For each cut or weave the boy made, the man matched him and, eventually, overcame the child and pinned him to the ground. We all stared, wondering if it was our place to intervene, a decision difficult to make since none of us knew the circumstances. Suddenly, Ibrahim appeared in the green Dodge Caravan and leapt out, inserting himself in between the two, forcing the pursuer to release his grip from the boy he had on the ground. The child was as scared as the man was upset. In language none of us understood, Ibrahim interrogated the man and boy. Both reacted to Ibrahim's involvement as a natural insertion of an authority figure into their dispute. After a minute or so, the man left satisfied and the boy's look of terror was gone. Only later did we find out that the cause of the melee was the boy extracting a measure of revenge against the man regards some familial dispute. The boy acted out his sense of justice by scaling the man's house wall and defecating openly in the courtyard, an act the man witnessed that set off the chase we witnessed. Ibrahim's fortuitous arrival may have saved the man from arrest, the boy from a serious beating and us from having to make a decision in a high stress situation about which we knew nothing. Without saying a word to us, Ibrahim calmly got back into his minivan to continue the morning's livery.

As Ibrahim drove us through the dark streets of Port Loko, I had only an image of red, gold and soccer balls, doing my best to crowd out the gnawing fear that I would be paired up next shift with a dilly dallying, time wasting partner again. Inside the compound, I went into the freezer and dug around the watery bottom, getting a mild shock as I fished out a water and a soda. 'Really should do something about that short,' I thought, too tired to really care enough. Out on the patio I drank my soda and then the water, watching the fruit bats fly in and out of the through-way of the building, snatching the bugs attracted to the lights. Finished up, I walked to my door, stepped over a sprawled out, sleeping Victor on the floor, and headed to bed, not even bothering to change out of my scrubs. Through my window, I could hear Ibrahim's minivan running before he turned it off, the van warm enough for him to lay down the seat for his nighttime bed. For a man who could someday be a chief, I thought, maybe he would have a better sleeping arrangement when that day came.

Big Stick

I took the limbless, barkless branch, a dozen feet long, and carried it inside to the donning tent and set it in the corner before I had to wrestle into my gear. Ali was plainly curious and asked, "What with that stick?" I turned around so he could spray down the soles of my boots and explained, saying, "I'm going to take it inside with me; there's something I can use it for," intentionally being vague.

"Hmm," Ali nodded, then looked down at my boots. "How long before you go home?"

"A little less than two weeks. Pretty anxious about these boots," I teased, going further, saying, "Well, maybe I really like these boots and want to take them home with me. What do you think of that?"

Ali lost his smile, frowning in disappointment. "But you promised..." then caught himself, trying to repeal any possible judgment by me of him being a common beggar.

I went too far, I thought, and then grabbed his black marker off his small desk. Sitting down on his watchman's chair, I untied my right boot and offered it up to him to see. Ali stood over me, watching, waiting to see what was next. Holding the toe of boot towards me, I took his marker and spelled out 'A-L-I' over the previous small 'ail', put the boot back on, then took the left boot and did the same.

"There," I pointed to the black lettering. "When I leave you get these boots. I won't forget."

Ali laughed and bumped my elbow, saying something in Krio that was likely complimentary if the grin on his face was any indication.

I rushed into the nurses' station and found my knapsack I had left from the night before, then just as quickly rushed out, hoping to avoid seeing anyone and being wrangled into doing some small task that would snowball into many and, before you'd know it, the day would be gone.

Two of the doctors cornered me the previous night, asking how I was feeling. Of course, 'everything's fine' is just the introductory sentence to every complaint ever aired. When I arrived home the previous night from the evening shift and had sacked out, I made the mistake of waking up and heading outside to scrounge up a snack off the lobby shelf. Both docs were out on the patio, up late, working their tablets. I joined them for some company and a chance to catch up on the latest.

'Everything's fine' wasn't satisfactory and the two of them ticked off the grueling cramp session I had two nights previous and that word got back to them I was not at all happy with Q. At first, I tried to set myself up as the fall guy, very unconvincingly proffering that I needed to take care of myself better and be more tolerant and flexible. One of the two docs immediately challenged me, saying, "You're not going to sit here and tell us that it was OK for you to be left inside for 5 hours handling all those admissions. Because it wasn't. I understand exactly how hard it is to walk away from what all of us consider important work and it's our fault we didn't do a better job of fortifying the schedule so that wouldn't happen."

I had no doubt that it was Mary who raised the issue since on the way home of that night I was basically furious. I left her at Dutch camp post shift and her attitude seemed oddly neutral. Either way, I had no expectation my physical well being, or the lack thereof precisely on that night, was going to be noticed. It's fairly memorable when someone is so disabled by muscle spasms they can't even sit up.

The second doc was listening intently, then asked, "How have the people assigned with you been?"

"They're really nice," I said with all sincerity. "Smart as hell. I like them." The answer was greeted with an obvious look of disbelief and a smirk.

"Well, we know Mary couldn't be with you because of the break in her skin and I personally know that Q can get bogged down in details that slow everyone down. I've worked with him. Brilliant doctor. Problem is, what makes him great in one place doesn't make him the best fit everywhere. We got a call from the nurse matriarch that one of the national nurses complained about you two being late in getting in and even later getting out. Would you say that's accurate?"

I paused. No one wants to throw anyone under the bus. One or two bad shifts is not a trend. My problems with Q's procrastination, though, were no longer just my own. The thinly manpowered schedule that devolved from adequate enough help being present at Maforki, to being a rice paper thin number of hands after some were bumped to the countryside to get outlying hospitals up and running, a move I felt was overly ambitious and ignored certain realities. We needed more help for the later shifts.

I let loose: the horrible condition of the patient stuck in the ambulance Joseph and I had tear out, how undignified and cruel it was; being inside the hot zone all those hours and missing meals over three days was an obvious set up for physical collapse; the two times I requested a meal be set aside, it was nowhere to be found, evidence to me of a lack of forethought. I complained Q had no sense of time, a habit that needed to be corrected immediately if he was going to avoid being persona non grata, as no one wants to waste time in an indefinite waiting pattern while he unpredictably scratches whatever curiosity nit he has. Last, I griped about the recent contract we were asked to sign, that we were agreeing we would all take one day off every seven, a giant exercise in denial that appeared to place the burden on the worker to set their schedule when in reality the peer pressure and undeniable need for everybody we could get was overwhelming. None of us had the power to write the schedule, further making an absurdity of the idea each person was in charge of their own day off.

The words spilled out. "If I have to sit around and wait two hours again where I have to do back to back rounds with time to only pee and get some water, I'll just appropriate a national nurse..." And so it went. I was on a roll.

Both of them were smiling. Maybe it was they agreed or maybe it was pathetically obvious I needed a rest after thirty some odd days as well as some real food.

"Your off tomorrow," the younger of the two smiled at me.

The pair caught me off guard but knew I was scheduled in, saying, "No, I have to go in at..."

She cut me off. "I know that. But you need the day off."

The second doc shook his head. "No doubt. And we'll talk to Q about being a little more punctual. Besides, he's been emailing people at 3 and 4 a.m. It appears he has no problem with a 24 hour day."

"Well," I huffed, "I do. There comes a point that a mind and body can only do so much without at least a change of routine or the ability to self direct. There's a huge difference between being able to complete tasks in your own way or having someone else dictate it without any knowledge of how it's going to happen or when it will be enough."

"Don't worry about showing up tomorrow," she firmly instructed. "You have anything fun you want to do?"

I wasn't sure whether to feel bad or good but decided quickly enough that a couple of good meals on schedule with everyone else would be a nice start. Then I laid out my plan how down by the river a young man offered to take me on a canoe trip in a dugout for a few bucks. Anything to do with water and wildlife would be a great diversion for me. "Yeah. Guided boat trip."

The both of them questioned me about the safety of it all and were satisfied that it was not risky or dangerous, wishing me the best. I thanked the both of them but in the back of my mind worried that maybe they thought I was 'the one who cracked'. No one wants to be that person. Then again, I hadn't missed a single round or went on any other type of assignment that might have served as well as a day off from the constant overarching battle with pestilence.

So now here I was at Maforki, trying to sneak out without being recognized or being wrangled for some errand. Outside the nurses' station, I put away down on the ground my large pole-stick for when I returned to work the next day. Just in case, I then checked the whiteboard to verify I wasn't assigned to any team. My eyes ran over the list of Cubans, nationals and Americans. And there I was: Team Two.

Inwardly I groaned, knowing I'd have to track down the team and explain why I wasn't going to part of their day. Fortunately, Carlos was one of the Cubans I had worked with previously and the second listed Cuban a couple of times, too. Normally, it was my job to get report on our assigned patients and more or less set a plan of action. I hopped over to the Cuban tent, loud with laughter as usual, and stood in the doorway, willing my own voice over the din. "Carlos!"

Carlos stood up. "Si!"

I waved him over and as best I could explain, told him I wasn't going to be with him, that he'd have to attend report and put together whatever he thought he would need for the day. He listened intently, arms folded, until I finished.

"No," Carlos said, shaking his head, continuing, "You come with us."

I wasn't prepared for any push back but in the short moment of panic that I was about to lose my day off, I found my resolve, saying, "Nope. You have to take the lead today. I'm not even supposed to be here." With that I turned, waving, and shouted, "Adios, Carlos! See you in the funny papers! Manyana!" I ran to the gate and out, nabbing a driver who was lingering outside, ordering him to get me back to the compound immediately. Off we sped, dodging the goats, pedestrians, dogs and motorcycles. The way he drove, you'd of thought it was his day off, too.

Back at the compound, I changed into a pair of hiking pants and light shirt. Back in the SUV, the new driver illustrated once again that his sense of urgency was greater than mine, speeding and weaving through the market circle and down to the Bankasoka River where Baker, my guide, was waiting as we had arranged earlier that morning.

Several days earlier Baker had stopped me on the way home from work as I was walking and inquired about a job. That was beyond what I could do but I asked if he knew anything about the river, how to get around on it. He did. His uncles fished it for a living and he would sometimes help. When I asked if he had access to a boat, he said that he did.

The unexpected day off worked out well for the two of us. Baker, all of 16 maybe, led us down a path to a mud flat with no less than a gaggle of kids following to see what the funny Apatow was going to do. One little girl of four kept popping up in the strangest places, wearing a princess crown fashioned out of stickers off of juice bottles. Her brown dress was neat and pressed with a pinned up personality to match. I gave her some mints that had been lying around my room, the child treasure equivalent of gold nuggets. No sooner than I had handed them out, on the sly so I wouldn't be mobbed by the other kids and disappoint because I didn't have enough, she was back in front of me asking for more. So again I gave her two more. This went on yet once again and I yielded the last of the mints. Baker laughed.

"What's so funny?" I asked.

He barked out something in Temne. In front of me, three little girls in brown dresses and home-made crowns of juice stickers lined up. Triplets. Identical triplets at that. Each smiling and giddy that they had bamboozled me out of the mints by pretending to be the same person, though I'm sure their plan took into consideration that the end result was a 2/3's less candy for what I thought was one person but that's not a flaw if identicals think of themselves as one entity.

Statistically, the sheer odds of three surviving identical triplets in such an impoverished country struck me as remarkable. The literature on multiple births puts the chances for identical triplets from anywhere between 1 in 60,000 pregnancies to one in 200 million. Even the most cautious bettor can probably say somewhere in between the two aforementioned figures lays the best answer if handled to put odds on it.

As the three of them stuffed their chubby cheeks, still laughing at having duped me, Baker came from down the bank dragging a narrow dugout canoe and settled it into the shallow water. With the tide low, I had to cross the mud for a few feet to get in.

I took the front of the rough dugout pirogue with Baker in the back. We both handled paddles and shoved off out onto the coffee colored water that was flat-perfect and unrippled, a mirror reflecting the blue sky and shoreline forest. Out on the water, larger boats that plied the river down to Freetown and the Atlantic ocean floated from net to net to check their catch. Baker explained that during the dry season wildlife congregated further down river, leaving fishermen with reduced harvests on this part of the river. The mango groves were thick with wintering white egrets of a variety I never was able to specifically identify. There was the occasional fish sunning itself as we passed over. They resembled something like a crappie you'd find back in Wisconsin or Minnesota. No hippos or crocodiles, but Baker did point out where, during the rainy season, crocs would crawl up on the islands to sun or nest, remnants of the muddy slide visible they created going in and out of the water on the banks.

After an hour or so we arrived at a village. Instantaneously, our pirogue was greeted by no less than 30 villagers of all ages, everyone shouting at once. They huddled Baker and me up the hill into the center of the village, a place with 20 or so thatched huts and not a speck of tin on any of them. Orange and plantain groves, interspersed with coconut trees, gave more than ample shade. One young boy decided he had to show off his tree climbing prowess and talent, scooching up 15 feet, gripping equally with his feet as his hands. Once at the top, he reached into a bundle of coconuts, twisted one off and tossed it to the ground. Back down from his tree, he handed the coconut to an elder who expertly macheted away the husk then split the nut into halves, creating natural cups to drink the juice. After we imbibed the juice, the white flesh was dug out in large flakes I could carry in my hand to snack on.

A low fire smoldered away with rice cooking in a large community pot. Plantains and oranges were heaped nearby. One old woman held a scrawny cat. I inquired if it was a pet and, as I suspected, it was not. No dogs were present.

With dogs so abundant and ubiquitous in Port Loko, this was out of place. Baker explained to me that not everyone was fond of dogs, and with the Ebola crisis, some people heard rumors of dogs at Maforki going in and out, thus dogs were no longer welcomed. Or maybe they just ate them all, Baker shrugged.

One of the boys brought out an old, beat up soccer ball, half deflated, and I was put out in the middle of a hardscrabble pitch where they showed off their skill of being able to dribble around me at will. With a little practice, I was soon enough able to pass accurately back and forth with each of the kids and not embarrass myself too much.

After the impromptu sports, the elder who cut up the coconut inquired if I had malaria medications or could get them, which, no, I could not. I apologized for being such an ineffectual, but Baker later assured me that many village chiefs who asked for malaria meds ended up selling them on the black market. And why not? What other source of income did they have to turn to when times became lean. A few packets of malaria meds might be enough to purchase a pig or a couple of goats, enough protein rich meat to feed a small village like this for a week or so. Yet, it is exactly this type of scenario many foreign governments consider corruption. Maybe the lens of scrutiny should be refocused to the circumstances, satisfied that the medication is getting into circulation at all.

The end of the visit had me palming 50,000 Leones into the blue and red fingernail polished hands of the village Papa that heightened my sense of guilt. Was I being some sort of patronizing slum tourist? I confided this to Baker as we headed back to the river, but he assured that if any others from my group wanted to visit the village, they were welcome. The money was always needed and the villagers enjoyed learning about the Apatow.

Back in the pirogue, we shoved off out onto the water. The tide was still receding, meaning we had a mild paddle against the current as well as the natural flow of the river. The stalled hydroelectric project bought the natural geography of the river some time, an asset in of itself. The down side was the delay of a large reservoir behind the dam that could be a reliable source of round the clock affordable electricity for industry, plus water which could also serve as a fishery, establishing a year round reliable local source of nutrition, commerce and occupation. Additionally, a reservoir would take pressure off the ground water wells that were susceptible to sputtering out as the dry season wore on, forcing more than a few families to rely on public water fountains that meant a serious amount of physical labor and time to get it back to home. Even more important, reliable water and electricity would be able to support a much more hygienic community, especially regards the local hospital, orphanages and schools. As it stood, a full standing shower was a luxury. The upside of the delay was no reservoir where malaria mosquitoes could breed.

Baker pointed out an anchored boat he sometimes worked with his two uncles, a fire engine red and yellow deep-hulled contraption of hand-hewn lumbers. He explained that his pair of uncles rented the hand tools needed to cut the best trees, sawyer the logs and finish each piece to size entirely by hand and by themselves. It was their first boat and they were working on a second as the dry season fish harvest was in its annual downturn he explained.

The immediacy between the land and the people has a stark presence unlike back in the States. At home, nearly every item of food in a household passes many hands and each item originates from a producer who specializes in one product, everything from strawberries to milk to meat are grown on farms and ranches devoted to one saleable product. Crops are sold and resold to packagers and canners and on to wholesalers and eventually retailers. The popularity of farmer markets is in no small part due to the immediacy between producer and buyer. Here, in Sierra Leone, this was the fabric of the way of life, i.e. you grew what you needed and sold the excess yourself, or you hunted or raised your own meat, first for you then, if extra, sold the excess. Back home, only one member of my own extended family still dairy farms. Here, everyone farms something or another. Here you have faith in your own ability to feed yourself, whereas back home you have faith in an entire infrastructure of fuels, transportation, markets, warehouses, buyers and sellers to deliver. I'm not sure which is more tenuous or reliable.

The lesson of simplicity is not lost on me regards this whole Ebola epidemic. How we were successfully treating patients with the scant resources we had versus how Ebola patients back in the states were treated, was as night and day as it could get. In the States, teams of nurses and docs focused on one patient, multiple lab samples drawn and swabbed to measure everything from electrolytes to blood cell counts. Neurological, GI and integumentary systems were observed and quantified likely as often as every 4 hours. Doctors entered orders into computers based on detailed patient examination, nursing notes, test results and the patient's reports. Unit clerks would verify orders, then nurses would again verify the orders, rectifying any discrepancies. The nurse would then divvy up the orders, noting which order applied to which specialist, be it doctor, phlebotomist, respiratory, dietary, nurses' aides, pharmacy and so on. Each day likely generated close to a 1/3 ream of paper for each patient. In the US, supplemental oxygen was probably an afterthought whereas here if a green tank of O_2 showed up, you could reasonably assume it was for some blacksmith shop's acetylene torch. Here a patient had a one sheet of paper bedside chart for every 6 days. In the States, patient records are measured in kilo and megabytes on servers that might be warehoused on the other side of the continent. When someone passes on, back in the States everyone from the newspaper, banks, insurance and credit card companies to tax collection agencies, coroners, funeral directors, town, city, county, state and federal agencies ranging from licensing boards to Social Security, get notified. Here, when one of the patients passed on, notification was mostly by way of a relative who inquired daily, usually in person, on the ill person's status and if they were in the Red Cross Death Book.

Back at our launch point, the kids were involved in their own games, the novelty of this Apatow not so novel anymore as they entertained one another rather than mawk for me and Baker. But as soon as they saw my camera come out, that all changed as they clamored for their personal and group portraits and to view the camera display.

I thanked Baker for his time and efforts, paid him and left, wondering to myself what his life would be like 10 years in the future. Barring some type of lottery-like break in the odds, his future was dictated by the draw of his birth. Sierra Leone is 6 million people and 27,699 sq. miles, a small place where, in part, size dictates available opportunities. Unless a Leonean was willing to surrender what meager advantages of native citizenship they had for a chance in another country, assuming they had the funds to even start an application process, and risk that money on a very uncertain approval, they were trapped. By comparison, someone in West Virginia, which is about 25,000 sq miles and 1.9 million people, can leave for 56 other states and territories that suit their talents and urban or environmental predilections. It's easy to shrug one's shoulders and say, 'Life isn't fair' as if solutions are beyond our capabilities and dictated completely by the fates, absolving us from even thinking about it. The reality is, life truly isn't fair and in no small part that it is due to manmade paradigms from government to access of capital and resources. Baker did not choose his paradigm, but others did. Baker can only change his circumstances when the others give him the permission to allow for freedom of movement. We humans are a jealous lot, not prone to share until we are certain of our own comfort; smart enough to know that competition truly does not make one better but that it risks losing what one has to someone else. No competition equals no competition. One less Baker in my bubble is one more of something for me, an easier way to get and keep. It is the essence of what drives so many Americans to spew vitriol over illegal immigration if you haven't already grasped the concept.

The triplet chubs made one appearance for me together then started a game of two running away and hiding, leaving one behind to finagle some sort of treat out of me. As they took each other's place and turn, it amused them to no end to think they were duping me. In that moment of time, it couldn't help but cross a person's mind that the whole point of the foreign presence was to enable these girls to keep laughing and playing.

Out past the mothers washing clothes in the river and up the gravel bank, the road was busy. Lockdown was finished and the routines of life were normalizing again. I put foot to blacktop and headed up hill through the market circle, past the government hospital, under the shade of the Kapok tree where Bernard the Ebola cemetery director and clan drank in the evening. Even the goats, dogs and chickens seemed to be in a brighter mood, more active and outgoing now that the lockdown was over. My own mood was as if someone drilled a hole in my head and let all the festering bile drain out, something I didn't even know was festering to begin with until it was gone.

Inside the compound, Tigger, on his pile of sand near the well, was oblivious to the world. On the patio table, a lunch had been saved and had my name on it, making me thank an absent Nolan profusely that likely did as much. I didn't understand how hungry I was until I ate, able to feel strength return to my body. Inside my room, peace and quiet put me into a slumber and dreams of white herons and water passed behind my eyes. Tomorrow was another day.

Big Stick Goes to Work

Over the next several days, admissions continued to pound the hospital. More hands were on the way but the problem was that almost as many would be leaving when they arrived. As we turned into more of a 24-hour operation, we were spread even more thin. Those assigned outreach duties in rural areas would pop in at times to lend a hand, a nice boost of help. The Cubans continued to be split into two 6 hours shifts, the British continued to tackle logistics and communications while the Dutch and Irish continued watching lots of soccer between lab runs and rural outreach.

On the first day back, the entire day shift crew was outside the admissions' building, mingling around stacks of clothing, food and mattresses, waiting for the discharge team to deliver the most recent survivors up to receive their food, bedding, clothes, Certificate of Health and ride home. The buzz in the group was that the last of the test results came back negative for the Kargbo uncle so the whole Josephine Kargbo family plus one agreed to leaving as one, just as Josephine insisted. In all, a dozen survivors were leaving upright and walking, immune to Ebola and now a national asset that could be enlisted to help fight the outbreak, though I'm not sure how much effort was actually put into maximizing that angle.

As soon as the outside the fence discharge team rounded the corner with the Kargbos, Josephine in her spotless white and gold dress and red jacket, others in a rainbow of bright shirts and lafas, everyone cheered and clapped. Smiles broke out, contagious. Anyone who had participated in the care stepped forward for the honor of a Josephine elbow bump, some ignoring the protocol and embracing each family member. Those not in the Kargbo clan were slightly off kilter by it all but eventually accepted the family triumph as their own, freely moving back and forth through the crowd to accept congratulations and best wishes. Soon, each had their name called out to put their own ribbon on the Survivor tree and be presented with their discharge gifts and paperwork. Photographs abounded.

When Josephine finished tying her own ribbon to the tree after those of her children, she raised both hands and brought them back down into folded prayer, proclaiming, "I never doubted God would deliver us from this evil and He did so by delivering us to you. Thank you. Thank you, God." The tears in her eyes finally came, tears of relief that those who came with her were leaving with her. Clasping arms tightly to demonstrate their commitment to the whole of the family, they stayed that way until they entered the van that would take them back to their home. Several of the national sprayers handled the Kargbo money and goods, making certain it was loaded and accounted for since none of the Kargbos appeared ready to relinquish their grasp of one another. The loss of any one of them, hopefully in a far off future, was going to be a profound loss in a way that would have never happened absent their collective experience of suffering the past 3 weeks.

Collective suffering from the ravages of a specific disease at the same time and place by an entire family are much rarer in the 21st century. When plagues and other communicable diseases left pockmarks on human history, communities suffered identically, communally. The advent of better treatments, mass vaccination programs and standardized hygiene has all but eliminated many epidemics, leaving disease to be much more of a personal trial and making illness socially distant. For many people, taking care of someone's medical needs is a rare event, now usually reserved for most of us to an immediate family member who is terminal or seriously disabled. Even then, professionals assume the more technical aspects through hospitalization, home visits and other medical and government support services.

For the staff, the victory of the Kargbos was a demonstration of proof that the odds were in the patient's favor. Ebola was still scary and to be respected but it was beatable, the survivor rate now just a tad over 70%

and holding steady. 80% or 90% was not out of the question, entirely realistic.

The celebration ended with everyone going back to putting themselves together for the first full round of the day. The rest of the day was uneventful in that nothing out of the ordinary happened. Deaths occurred and bodies transported to the morgue. Some patients improved while others lingered on the fence and could go either way. Staff continued to do as much as they could with what was available. Even a crisis has a routine when it goes on long enough.

The next few days, admissions held steady and acuity levels as a whole were stable. The outlying centers were set up and beginning to open, closer to the hotspots of where the Ebola outbreak was being more tenacious. One would think that the slums of Freetown would be more problematic but when a million people are rubbing elbows, news travels fast and response times for quarantined treatment and contact tracing are much quicker thanks to the very proximity that also enables the spread of a disease. In rural areas, people are more spread out and able to hide their illness much better. Some would wander into the bush to die or seek out the only known medical treatment, a traditional medicine man or woman, oblivious to the threat they faced personally and posed to their own small villages. The hope of the aid organizations was to educate the populace in proper preventive hygiene practices, to report all deaths and refrain from secretly treating or burying the sick, something many secret societies did with their ill or deceased members.

Even though total infections in the country continued to climb, the rate of new infections slowed and Maforki ETU held steady, all evidence that the new outreach was beginning to take hold. It was January now and one day I met a man who introduced himself as a Sierra Leonean doctor who would be heading up the contact tracing training of nationals. This caused me to perk up my ears. I had assumed that the contact tracing teams were largely composed of Sierra Leoneans with foreign aid workers interspersed within the effort. We were now over a year into common knowledge of the outbreak and 8 months into the epidemic and still at this late date, the country did not have charge of the contact tracing.

I had a poor position from which to grasp an overview of the world response, how it unfolded and was organized. The most apt metaphor would be me at the bottom of a well, able to look up and only deal with what was in front of me. What exactly others were doing outside of the well was revealed in pieces of generalized email memos and informal conversations. By comparison, the 2010 earthquake in Haiti, getting people from various nongovernmental organizations to work together amounted to an exercise in futility due to the lack of a top down structure that could survey each organization's talents and assign the right aid group to the right job in the right place. Much of the money pledged was slow in coming and what money was made available quickly was often eaten up by the aid organizations themselves back in their home base countries, dedicated to logistics of getting people into Haiti. One figure I read claimed that only 10 cents on the dollar reached an actual Haitian who needed housing, clothing, food or medical care. Some reports claimed it was even less.

One instance of misplaced resources during the Ebola outbreak was the erection of hospitals in neighboring Liberia by the US Army. President Obama managed to finagle promised billions from a reluctant US congress for the US Army to organize and deploy 4,000 soldiers to erect the hospitals in Liberia, but the drawback was the uniqueness of the response needed and the location, something that required weeks of planning. After 4 months, though, the US Army had the hospitals up in Liberia but by that time, Liberia, in co-operation with NGO's, managed to extinguish the worst of their Ebola outbreak. Beautifully built and wonderfully clean, climate controlled units went unused and sat empty. Liberia's saving grace was a stronger central government that had a history of strong and organized co-operation with NGO's in-country, logistical infrastructure in place that facilitated a more rapid and organized deployment of skills and resources to where it was needed. Sierra Leone, a country twice as poor as Haiti, was anarchy by comparison.

I know some of my colleagues were deeply involved in cobbling back together what was left of the overall clinical infrastructure in Sierra Leone, the goal being something predictable and reliable to be in place to help the country deal with the everyday medical needs of the population. Lack of funds, talent and supplies is an understatement, implying that there were systems in place to properly manage the aforementioned should they become available. Entire algorithms and hierarchies needed to be invented. Was this the wise use of resources at the time? I personally could make an argument against such a use, the analogy being that you shouldn't start ordering lumber for the new house until the forest fire that incinerated it is out. Others felt that a basic, reliable clinical structure would be receptive to being ramped up in times of crisis and that since we were already present, now was the time to strike that bargain.

My schedule eventually shifted back into evenings with my last two days being on nights before my term was up. With the arrival of several new nurses and doctors, evening shift was no longer a lone sentinel position, two full teams able to divide things.

Dr. Dahna and I were assigned together for my last night shift. We crawled into the complex at near midnight and took report from the evening shift. Any ideas we had about a quiet shift evaporated as we went over the patient report with the departing shift. Two infants were unable to be cared for by their mothers, needed IV's and to be fed by us. The same went for several toddlers. Other patients were showing signs of delirium, suffering either from meningitis or hypernatremia, a sodium imbalance, and wandering off outside or frightening the other patients. They would likely need their IV's restarted since they had pulled out what IV access they had. On it went. It was just us, the patients and dogs.

Dr. Dahna and I headed over to the nurses' station and we put together an inventory of what we thought we would need, drew up our syringes and bagged everything else. All the sprayers were asleep and the national nurses were quiet, a peaceful respite from the constant daytime noise of boom boxes and chatter.

As we gathered up our gear, Dahna asked, "Are you going to miss it at all?"

I looked at her, not sure how to answer, and then said, "I'll miss the people we work with. Will I miss the work itself? Maybe. But I'm happy that I was given the chance to do it."

Finished suiting, we checked each other over and went down together to rouse a sprayer from his sleep, knocking quietly. A young man named Jon came out, explaining he wasn't the assigned sprayer but wanted to go in place of the other fellow, that it was OK.

I shrugged. "Fine. We're ready to go."

Jon made haste and packed his tank. I grabbed my boots from outside the nurses' station and spotted the big stick I had brought in a week earlier, and grabbed that, too. Away to the inside we went. Jon, rather than following as the sprayers usually did, led instead, saying, "We'll start with Suspect 1 and follow through. I know at least one of the patients will need Paracetamol and fluids."

Jon led us inside and put down his tank, immediately heading to the table where the meds were, digging through the grab bag of packets until he came up with what he was looking for. He popped the packs for what he wanted and proceeded to assist the patient to take an antipyretic and then hung a fresh bag of IV fluids, setting the drip rate.

Dr. Dahna looked over our patient we were tending, saying, "Nurses shouldn't have to be double as sprayers on night shift. Have they always done it?"

I shook my head 'no', then said, "A couple of times one of the nurses would tell the sprayer to get some sleep instead, that it made no sense to have a sprayer on the slow night shifts. It works out OK."

Dahna finished off the bedside notes and we continued on outside to Suspect 2 where all was quiet and dry, leaving us to only record temps and jot readings in the notes. Out we went with Jon leading the way to Suspect 3. He stopped on the doorstop, turning to us, saying, "There are a mother and infant in here who are doing very poorly. I'll take care of the mother if you two take care of the infant. OK?"

"No problem," Dr. Dahna agreed.

Jon turned on the light and illuminated the worst of things, diarrhea and vomit puddling on the floor, half-eaten food intermingled. One young man was staring up at the ceiling, eyes wide and bulging, mumbling. His pants were off and he was only half on his mattress. I kneeled on the concrete and sat the poor soul up, then pulled the mattress underneath him as Dr. Dahna and Jon each took one of his arms and lifted him. Likely meningitis. I stood up.

"You have stool on you," Dahna pointed to my left arm, brown juice dripping off my elbow. Jon pumped the chlorine pack and sprayed me down.

"Is it gone?" I asked.

Both agreed it was taken care of.

Down in the corner beneath a cholera bed, a mother and infant were lying, eyes half open on the both of them. Mother was curled up, on her side on one end, and the infant was on the other end, naked and uncovered, exposed to the cool night air, bluish white, startlingly Caucasian looking in its complexion.

"Is this a black child?" I asked Dahna.

She picked up the infant and held it out at arm's length to get a better view under the fluorescent lights, educating me, saying, "It probably has low iron. Melanin formation needs iron. Probably the baby has a low red count." She then pulled the infant into her bosom to warm it. It made no sound at all.

Jon fiddled with the mother's IV. As he was hooking the line for a fresh bag, the fellow we had put full on the mat prior, was on his feet, stumbling blindly towards Jon. With our backs towards the action, none of us saw him until it was too late. Dahna jumped back off to the side to get herself and the infant out of the way, spilling formula and pediatric acetaminophen syrup over herself and the baby. I reached out to grab the bumbling patient, getting a piece of his shirt in my hand, It wasn't enough and he tripped on Jon's legs, crashing down on the floor, hitting his head on the concrete. It sound something like an over ripe tomato being hurled against a wall. He then rolled over, his eyes as wide open as when we came in, speechless.

Jon was knocked on his rear-end and the mother remained oblivious, not flinching. Jon looked around the floor, then asked, "Do you see the syringe?"

Dr. Dahna and I stepped closer, scanning the ground and under the beds. No syringe.

"Here," I said to Jon, getting down on the floor with him and grabbing our crashing wanderer by the shoulders, saying, "I'll roll him towards me. Maybe he's on it."

I rolled the patient towards me and put him up on his side. As soon as I did, a stream of bloody diarrhea began flowing out, a black-brown blood infused sewage spreading over the floor. Jon reacted but not as I expected, nearly shouting, "Syringe!", holding it up in victory. Dahna grabbed a handful of rags and threw them on the demented man's mess. It was no use moving him off the mess since it would likely only be moving him to make more messes. The three of us decided that it was easier to drag the mother and infant's mattress to the empty corner across the room. We did this and covered the man, choosing to focus on the mother and infant.

Jon was quietly talking to the mother and attempting to get her to drink some fluids along with some oral meds of one sort or another. Dr. Dahna and I focused on the infant, she holding him while I drew up some more formula and acetaminophen into a syringe. Dr. Dahna brushed the infants lips, attempting to solicit the latching reflex as I put the syringe tip over the infant's mouth and tried to dribble in the solution. The infant would push its tongue once or twice, stop, and then start to nod off.

"Come on, little guy," Dr. Dahna coached. She would give the infant a small wobble and brush his lips again as I tried to dribble some of the medicated formula into the child. Again, the infant would push his tongue once or twice as if he was interested but again he would nod off, his eyes drifting shut.

We did this three or four more times with no success other than spilling a good amount of formula onto the baby. Dr. Dahna wrapped the child in a few large fresh rags and placed it in the crook of the mother's waist. Mom didn't react at all other than to squint her eyes and close them again. Patients this quiet tend to be in the throes of severe pain, hoping that lying still will not aggravate the problem.

"Cover them with this," Jon directed, handing us a clean brown surplus blanket to throw over the pair. Dr. Dahna made a pillow of some rags and positioned the baby near the mother's head, then covered the pair.

Across the room in another corner, an older female patient began lecturing us, her words unintelligible. "What's she saying, Jon," I asked.

"I don't know," Jon shook his head. He turned to the med table and fished into our red bag and pulled out a syringe, asking, "Is this Valium?"

Dahna looked at the dosage and acronym in black marker she had put on it, confirming, "Yeah, it is. Why…." And before she could ask why Jon wanted to know, he took three strides to the patient who was now trying to get off the bed, unsteadily at that, and took her under the arms to lower her to the floor. No small feat since she was bigger than Jon. Once on the floor, he readied the syringe by carefully pulling the safety cap, saying, "This is to help you get some rest."

Dahna and I looked at each other, watching Jon set up the shot. He placed his left hand on the woman's hip, fingers spread as a V and with his right hand thrust the needle between the two sets of fingers.

"Christ! What the hell you doing?" I shouted. "Are you trying to stick yourself?"

Dr. Dahna aired her bewilderment with less vehemence, asking, "Jon, are you a nurse or a nursing student?"

With confidence, even maybe a tinge of pride, Jon explained, "I want to go to nursing school. I watch all the doctors and nurses very closely. I'm learning the words and the drugs and why. I read the drug books and the books on disease."

I sensed he wanted us to admire this ambition. Then I remembered. At least twice I had been over at the admissions building and saw this young man at the desk reading and asking who ever would pay attention how to pronounce certain medical terms or drug names. A curious fellow in at least two senses of the word. Now here he was, practicing medicine. And, man, he needed the practice.

Dr. Dahna looked at me and asked, "I thought he was a nurse."

"I did to," agreeing with her.

He arranged the patient on a mattress on the floor and covered her with a blanket then, without hesitation, moved on to the next patient, taking the bedside chart and reading it over, checking the temperature and giving some Paracetamol, metoclopromide and diazepam followed by hanging a fresh IV bag.

I bumped Dahna to get her attention, asking, "Should we be letting him do this?"

"Technically, no," she laughed, then she stepped over next to Jon, interrupting him. I joined the pair.

"You aren't supposed to do this," Dahna gently warned Jon. "But we're going to use you." Dr. Dahna asked if I was OK with that and I was. She laid out the ground rules, made Jon demonstrate that he knew how to read a medication administration chart and quizzed him about dosages and the major pitfalls of the medications we administered. The most basic rule was that he had to read the bedside chart and explain to us what he was going to do before doing it and that we must be no more than one bed away. And no needles. His enthusiastic agreement was as if we just graduated him from school. On we continued.

Things had started out not so badly, meaning the patients were generally responsive. In Suspect 3, the patient with suspected meningitis or some sort of cerebral encephalopathy was disconcerting, us not knowing what he'd do next. Him smashing his head into the concrete was ominous and gut wrenching, something that back home would trigger an investigation and a plethora of tests to ascertain any possible damage. Here we couldn't even manage basic safety restraints or put a sentinel on him to guard him against further harm.

Dr Dahna returned to the infant and one more time we tried to coax the child into taking some medicated formula but had the same result as earlier. The infant would wake with a light rub but nod back off, eyes slowly taken over by sleep. Oddly enough, the temperature was about normal, indicating no infection but the bluish tinged lips, very pale complexion and undetectable femoral pulse pointed towards likely internal hemorrhage. Yet the whites of the eyes were clear. It was hard not to conclude that the infant was in shock or going into shock.

"He's dying," Dr. Dahna concluded. "Should we try an IV?"

My first thought was it was too late but I decided to back her up.

"I suck at pediatric IV's like this. You're going to have to take the first attempts," I said, hiding behind her superior training.

Jon was messing around at the table, apparently listening to us. He shouted for our attention, holding up a small package with something green in it. "Is this what you need?" he asked, stepping closer and showing us.

"An IO," Dr. Dahna exclaimed. "Problem solved, guys."

Jon was holding a pediatric interosseous screw port. Dr. Dahna took the package and unwrapped it, checking to make sure it was small enough to fit the need. Deftly, as if she did it more than a few times, she went over the infant's sternum and marked her spot, first pressing down to go through the skin then screwing it into the bone. Blood dribbled back exactly as it should. Jon had an IV line ready and I grabbed a bag of fluids. In a few seconds, normal saline solution was steadily and predictably trickling through the drip chamber. Dr. Dahna slowed it to a fast drip. After several minutes, she checked the femoral pulse, proclaiming it was definitely easier to find but that it was bradycardic, slow.

"Look at the chest," Dr. Dahna pointed out, continuing, "The respirations are too slow, too shallow. He probably has no red count worth anything. How much fluid has he gotten so far?"

Jon put his face up to the bag. "About 200, 250 cc."

"Stop it," Dahna ordered.

I clamped the line off and Dr. Dahna unhooked it. She then unscrewed the IO port and taped a bandage over the baby's sternum. Next to no blood showed, likely meaning there was poor blood pressure and too little blood to perfuse the tissues at a healthy level. Despite about 200cc of saline solution, it was doing nothing to prevent circulatory collapse.

Through all this, the infant's eyes continued the same pattern, opening with some physical stimulation but drifting back shut when it stopped. Jon bought over an empty IV fluids box and broke it down to make a crib. Dr. Dahna wrapped the child in fresh clean rags and covered him with a blue-green lafa, settling the box back down near the mother.

Dr. Dahna leaned into the mother, softly whispering through her mask and visor, apologizing, "I'm so sorry." The mother, not flinching, but with raspy voice over her cracked lips, replied, "Thank you," and closed her eyes.

Jon checked the mother's IV and asked if he should give her some Paracetamol, maybe some Valium. Dr. Dahna instructed him to administer 10mg Valium rectally and the same for 1000 mg Paracetamol, enlisting me to help if needed. Surprisingly, he didn't flinch, managing to get all four tablets well placed into the rectal vault as my digital check revealed. The mother was in no shape to take anything orally.

We finished Suspect 3, covering as many patients as we could with blankets against the cool night then exited, turning out the lights. All three of us knew that the infant would not likely be alive at sunrise. Possibly the mother as well. We didn't even have a PCR result as yet to inform us if we were dealing with Ebola or malaria.

If Suspect 3 had its sad stories, Suspect 4 greeted us with angry patients. As we went bed to bed, everyone was soaked in diarrhea. One patient was deceased long enough that rigor mortis had set in. The anger was palpable enough that I worried about retaliation of some sort. Jon immediately began engaging the patients in their native tongue, apologizing. Dr. Dahna and I gathered up as many clean clothes, rags and lafas as possible and started, one patient at a time, to clean them up and medicate for comfort. Jon left the building and returned with a body bag the three of us laid out to roll the corpse into, zipping it shut. Jon sprayed it and us down. He and I each took a side and carried the body out onto the gravel courtyard then laid it down to catch our breath. We decided we would muscle it the next 100 yards or so to the morgue, which we did, going slow to avoid tripping on the scattered brush and sticks. I couldn't help think this was a little like how early 18th century anatomists operated, under cover of darkness scavenging graveyards and purloining corpses for their forbidden studies.

We met Dahna outside the door of Suspect 5. The three of us now had been in for over an hour, the majority of the round still in front of us.

"Everyone fine?" I asked.

Both nodded, and with determination pressed on into S-5. More of the same, but worse. Not only were the patients upset but two of them were upset and delusional, cerebral encephalopathy likely taking hold.

At least three had yanked out their IV's. When Dr. Dahna and Jon tried to convince them of the wisdom of placing a fresh one, they refused.

"They do not trust us," Jon translated. "They think it's poison."

"Why do they think that?" Dr. Dahna asked, exasperated.

Jon spoke to what seemed the most lucid patient who kept pointing to a corner as they spoke. Jon finished and explained, "That man told them it was no good. That our medicine is a trick, that it's poison." Then Jon, too, pointed to the corner the patient had pointed towards.

I walked over to the shadowy corner and when I was close enough, I saw who the misinformant was. With not a little disgust, I remarked, "You. I thought you'd be gone." I grabbed the bedside chart to check the admit date and notes. I was right.

The patient misinforming and frightening others in S-5 was the same fellow delivered via ambulance a week earlier exhibiting clear signs of mental illness, acting out severe paranoia and possibly audio and visual hallucinations. He was the one that kept blocking my attempts to scan his temperature, who frightened other patients enough that they left the building minutes after we bedded him. Now, instead of frightening anyone, he somehow managed to capture his fellow patients' confidence enough to be taken at his word. Exhibit A was the corpse lying amongst them to bolster his argument.

I turned to Jon. "Tell the rest of the patients not to listen to this man. We aren't part of any curse," I said, feebly trying to defend us.

Jon engaged the man, who refused to look Jon in the eye, then would only mumble back responses that, for practical purposes, were incoherent. Jon became more animated and emphatic but the man only retreated further into his corner, becoming less responsive. Finally, Jon quit arguing, turning away in disgust.

"He insists we are the reason for the sickness," Jon explained, repeating what we already knew.

"Why is everyone else listening to him?" Dahna asked, continuing, "It's obvious he's not in his right mind."

Jon then deadpanned why. "He claims to be a medicine man. You don't question the medicine man."

And that was it. The rest of the patients were not only satisfied with the unstable man's explanations for the reasons for their illness, they were more or less obligated to respect his authority.

We decided to continue with the assigned cares, trying to perform assessments and administer medications. To a person, they refused to allow themselves to have their temps scanned and refused fresh IV starts. The refusal even extended to encouragement to take oral medications and drink from the 1.5 liter water bottles we handed out to them. Most bottles were untouched.

"This is a disaster, Doc," I observed. "If they aren't dehydrated from diarrhea and throwing up, refusing to take IV's and drinking will do it for them."

"All we have to do is convince them one of us is a stronger medicine man," Dahna offered matter of factly, as if it was obvious and was probably taught the first day of medical school.

"When's that going to happen?" I asked, the doubt in my voice clear.

"Day shift," Dahna said, nonchalantly passing the torch on this one. An excellent choice.

Being able to assert a plausible authority and trust when you're dressed as Anonymous is a tough sell. As Americans, our history is an open book with enough factual fodder for any pro-con argument about intentions. The few minutes of contact each day wasn't go to persuade those who were firm on any idea about us. I was never able to gauge how that level of trust or distrust affected other nationalities like the Cubans, though I think they flew under the radar just as their profile in the world might be described.

We finished in S-6 and prepared to move on. I backtracked to the fence where I put my stick and tried not to be spotted with it as Dr. Dahna and Jon moved on ahead of me. The dark of the night was adequate for me to bring the bare stick to the separating gate and toss it over as the pair entered into C-3. It landed on the stones with a rattling clunk.

Inside C-3, the first patients to our left quietly lay on two mattresses on the floor, a mother with a toddler of about 3 years and on the other a brother and sister, around 5 and 6. There was no enthusiasm or discontent on their part regards our arrival. Quietly, we went over the bedside notes and Jon gathered up as-needed medications as Dr. Dahna instructed while I checked temperatures and other signs. Empty bags of saline and IV antibiotics littered the surrounding floor along with untouched food.

Dahna checked over the mother and toddler, trying to encourage formula into the child while Mom completely surrendered involving herself, the weight of her sickness crushing her into the mattress. On my knees, I removed the blanket covering the boy and girl, greeted by the boy rubbing sleep from his eyes. Trying to be reassuring, I patted him on the shoulder with my gloved hands and patted his makeshift pillow of rags to assure him he could continue to try to sleep. Instead, he sat up.

Then he began speaking to me in Temne, quietly trying to have me understand. I could not. I ran the thermometer's red beam across his temple and it displayed the expected result that he was running a fever. Jon had put a bottle of pediatric pain reliever between Dr. Dahna and me so I poured 25 mls into the cup and motioned for the boy to take it. He pushed it away only to have me push towards him again and he conceded to swallow it. Again, he began pleading with me.

"He's asking about his sister," Jon translated.

"OK," I replied, not sure what to tell the boy.

I ran a thermometer scan across the apparently sleeping child. 34.4 C. I did a quick conversion in my head. About 94 F. Then I watched her chest. In the dim fluorescent light it was difficult to ascertain how much of the bluish hue of her complexion was the lights or was her. The boy tugged my arm but I held my hand up to signal for him to wait then put the same hand on her chest, then neck, to assess breathing and pulse. Through the gloves, I could feel the abnormal coolness incompatible with life. The boy, still sitting up, was more animated, distressed, repeating the same over and over. Jon began speaking to him, trying to be reassuring. The mother would open her eyes briefly then close them as Dr. Dahna continued working the 3 year old.

"Deceased?" Dr. Dahna asked.

"I'm afraid so," I quietly said. No one else said anymore. Even the boy stopped speaking, instead intently watching our next moves.

Looking around the building, I didn't see any unused blankets or clean lafas to wrap the girl. Even if a body bag was available, I would not have used it, the situation morbid enough without the sterile vinyl being unfolded and laid out. I stood up and walked the perimeter of C-3, hoping I would find a spare blanket. Several beds over, a younger looking man was watching, wrapped snugly into his blanket against the January night chill.

As I was prepared to continue walking past him, he tossed the blanket off his shoulders, sat himself up and grunted at me, holding the blanket out. I hesitated to accept one of the few comforts he had but he pointed towards the floor where he had his bundle. In it was a heavy winter coat. I took out the winter jacket, one like you'd find on just about anyone living in Buffalo, and we exchanged.

I went back to the mattress and covered the girl but not before I folded her dead arms back into her chest and rolled her back onto the spread out brown wool. Her eyes had begun to dry, the brown irises starting to look cloudy, half-covered by eyelids that would neither stay shut nor open. I wrapped the blanket over the feet, then head, and scooped my arms underneath, lifting her and myself off the floor.

Jon covered the barely audible moaning boy with what was no longer a shared blanket and laid him down, speaking gently. As I came to the door, I turned sideways and caught the boy looking, his red eyes melting with grief that no tears would cool. He never cried out.

C4 was empty due to efforts to consolidate patients and make rounds a bit quicker for everyone who served them. The only beds were cholera beds with their hole in the center. The girl's length was such that my placing her towards the head of the bed was adequate. Jon followed me with the spray pack and took the first step of the decontamination process, unfolding the blanket and misting over the body, then recovering and misting the blanket itself. We turned out the lights, leaving her for the eternal night that snatched her.

Back in C-3, Dahna busied herself at the remaining beds, jotting notes and administering medications. By the boy's mattress, I saw three empty blister packs of oral diazepam that were not present when I left. Mother, boy and toddler now had their two mattresses smashed together, sharing one blanket. The blanket the boy and girl shared just moments ago, was tossed onto the concrete several feet away.

We hurried our pace, wading through the swill, pleas and dogs, having been inside too long. Everyone needed a break, something to eat and drink. At the doffing station we had to yell to the outside to wake up a doffing sprayer, holding us up another 15 minutes. Eventually, the three of us got out, the night air raising goose flesh on our dripping moist skin.

At the nurses' station Dr. Dahna scratched out some notes she would pass on at morning meeting. Names on the whiteboards would be rearranged. All three of us exchanged wet scrubs for fresh, instantly warmer ones we packed with us but still needing wraps of our own to ward off the graveyard shift chill.

The only sound was the steady whine of the generator, a literal night and day difference on the ears. Jon slumped in a corner, napping, while Dahna tapped away at some keys on her laptop, hoping to eke out some unread emails. Above me, a hand sized moth with wings that had broad, deep, string-like borders, the rest of the wings scaffolded with fine, pink veins of spider web like threads. A slow curve of horn with a swell of yellow extended off the back of each wing. The moth would slowly pump its wings once or twice then become motionless as it clung to the fluorescent lights.

Off the top of a filing cabinet, I grabbed the notes for C-3 and began paging through, taking in the names, dates of admission and latest PCR results. Some of the patients are gone, discharged or deceased, but no one removed their note, or for those who were still present, the notes had not been reconciled for a couple of days. The only reliable aspect of the notes was that they were evidence someone tried to remember something about the persons inside.

I found the name I was looking for: Mariatu Sesay, 5 years age. Mother Kadiatu Sesay. Brother and sister Ali Sesay, 7, and Alicia Sesay, 3 years. All four were Ebola positive and self admitted.

Would Kadiatu have driven her family through our gates if she had any idea what was inside? If she knew how the dogs' toenails clicked on concrete in the dark of the night; the violent flatulence, sour rot and wretching; how some of the patients would stare right through each other as if they already no longer existed. All that can be said, is some were merely present while others suffered a grueling metamorphosis of the mind that robbed them of the innate and cultivated sense of self. So many had become abandoned ruins.

Ali. 7. What was I doing when I was seven? Sitting cross-legged on the green carpeted floor of my family's small town home, watching Walter Cronkite narrate the Apollo missions as they circled the moon. I even could recall the Christmas mission where one of the astronauts read the Creation Story from the Book of Genesis. I was warm, fed and well. All of our game farm animals of ducks and pheasants were bedded and fed. My parents dying or a brother dying? Inconceivable. You had to get old for that.

94 F. Covered in a heavy wool blanket with her brother spooning her to keep her warm. Ali must have thought he was doing a brotherly thing, that his sister, Mariatu, was in a peaceful, pain free deep sleep. He had his head nuzzled into her neck, arms across her torso when we arrived. 94 degrees. She was likely gone for three or four hours, Ali's body heat slowing the cooling of Mariatu's corpse.

My first inclination was to remove Mariatu's page to keep the binder uncluttered, a problem where other patients had passed but no note recorded and the page left in, misleading and confusing for anyone who was hoping for good information. I found the other 3 pages for Ali, Kadiatu and Alicia and sandwiched Mariatu's note just beneath her mother's ahead Ali's, then put all four names on each of the four pages to alert they were a family. If I tossed Mariatu's page, likely it would be hauled to the fire pit. I forced myself to imagine Ali watching me do such a thing.

I closed the binder and put it back on the file cabinet. My 6 weeks at Maforki was down to three hours left. The three of us folded up, arms crossed and chins on our chest, napping, thinking. The next thing I felt was a nudge, Dr. Dahna pushing my foot with hers.

"You going back in?" she asked.

I gathered myself and stood up to stretch. "Yeah. How about you?"

"I'm going to do a quick round with the morning nurse. There's not really much to do except hang some fresh bags. I just want to make a current report at morning rounds." Dhana then began prepping.

Jon peeled a plantain.

I looked at Dr. Dahna, saying, "I'm going to take Jon in with me. This is my last time. There's something I want to take a look at before I leave."

Whether she was tired herself or thinking five steps ahead, I don't know. But she didn't object, saying, "Me and the morning nurse are just going to lay eyes on everyone. That's fine."

I stepped outside and looked east. The telltale first purple and orange of dawn was giving way to gold and yellow, lighting things up enough that some of the solar night lights were flickering out.

"Hey, Jon, come in with me," I prodded.

Chewing the last of his plantain, mouth half-full, "What for?"

I explained about why I had taken in the big stick. To my surprise, he was ambivalent but decided to humor me, compromising, telling me he would go in through the gate back by the showers and meet me at the fire pit whenever I was ready. Then the two of us went into the donning tent and prepared.

I went through the gate into Suspect, on through Confirmed, to find my stick. This gate was one-way. They're all one-way. Each door opened up to an increasingly throat tightening set of deteriorating problems. It's not fair to use a Dante's 'Inferno' analogy; his is fiction. I grasped the stick and checked it over for snags, nails or anything else that could tear a glove, satisfied it was OK. It was getting lighter but no one inside or outside was stirring. Soon enough they would be.

I ducked between C-1 and C-2 and towards the back, the palm trees and bush brushed in violet by the low morning light. Jon was waiting in the low corner near the gate by the showers.

"I want to poke around in the old fire pit," I said, gesturing with my stick.

"Well, there isn't a new a fire pit anymore," he joked. The new pit was a heap of blackened tin roof panels on top of sooted up cinder blocks. Images of ACME company products and the Road Runner came to mind.

We both looked into the old pit, anything smoldering from the day before had burned itself out, though the acrid smell of burnt garbage was present. The cinder block wall surrounding the pit was maybe 2 feet high, low enough for me to kneel and work through the rough lumber railings.

"Hang on to me," I instructed Jon, extending my right arm for him to hook into and steady me. There was no real chance I was going to tumble in, but on the off chance that I would be overcome by smoke or somehow screw things up enough to start going over the side, he might be able to pull me back.

Looking in at the debris, it was impossible to assess how far down the bottom was. On the surface, there were only partially burned bags of waste, while in the deeper spots it was more ashes as each layer was incinerated day to day. I jammed all 10 feet of stick down, having only about 16 inches at the top for my hand to grasp.

With each prod, an echo would telegraph up the stick, varying between snappy for solid, rocky ground at the bottom; hollow thuds for old, partially burned buckets; soft for collisions with clothes and paper products. Where there were ashes, the stick would push through easily at first, then take more muscle to get it to the pit bottom. After two or three minutes of this, I could tell the difference, visually checking myself to see if what I was feeling was what I could see. There was enough daylight to illuminate, the rising sun reflecting off the underside of the tin roof down into the pit.

Jon remained wordless as we moved foot by foot along the edge. Both of us were warming up. I continued jamming the stick, confident I had mastered the feel of the different items, a macabre sort of Braille. What bags were unburned were easy to move, mostly filled with Styrofoam, plastic water bottles and our old white suits. All the light colored stuff was moist enough to keep the fires to a low smolder, the smell and haze permeating the unit every day.

After twenty minutes, I had covered quite bit of ground, probably more than two thirds using a grid pattern where I probed a square foot or so then moved on to the next square foot in linear, methodical fashion. Then I plunged the staff once yet again just like one hundred times before and felt ash, then something like a rubbery substance with a woody interior. I pushed again until the stick stopped, noticing a slight rebound of the stick when my grip was loosened.

Without any prompting, Jon remarked, "That sounds different."

I shook my head in agreement. Jon let go of me and took to his knees next to me to get a better look. Both of us peered through the floating ash that had been stirred up, able to see enough to make out colors, shapes and objects. Most of what we could make out was white suits, clear plastic bottles with blue labels, melted Styrofoam meal containers, office paper, discarded clothing and lafas. The majority of what was on top towards the end of the pit we had already surveyed, yet to be fully burned. Where the stick was going now was definitely mostly ash, the lesser used receiving end of the pit the last few days that had managed to burn itself down.

"How far through the ash do you think we're going?" I asked Jon.

I slowly dropped the stick until the probe end was touching the top of the ash, then we watched how far it went until the bottom was signaled.

"Half meter," Jon guessed.

"Yeah," I agreed.

I continued to probe around the spot of interest, trying to eliminate any false alarms that might mimic what we found earlier. I handed the probe over to Jon and had him get a feel by poking and pushing in various spots we had covered so we could put our heads together.

"Now go back to that spot right there, where I was," I pointed, further instructing, "about three feet towards us away from that clump of melted water bottles."

Jon slowly pushed and pulled the probe in the approximate spot, calling out, "Ash," with each new move. Then, "Definitely not ash. I don't think it's any other garbage, either."

Jon now moved the stick side to side, covering just a few inches either way before being satisfied he was back in ashes.

"Go the other way. Length ways," I instructed.

Jon made short jabs until he found the spot again and moved up about a foot or so before remarking he was in ash again. Reversing direction, he made short jabs for about 4 feet before obviously being in ash again.

I took the stick from him and levered through the ash until it stopped against something soft I could rock, but not overturn whatever it was. Jon took a turn again, doing the same, then started stirring the ash as much as possible off whatever it was we were up against. Ash dust plumed up, obscuring our vision but he kept going, then ceased. We waited for the dust to settle.

"What do you think it is?" I asked Jon, knowing his answer.

"I think it's him." The disappointment in his voice was near grief.

After a couple of minutes, most of the dust had cleared and both of us looked back down. The light was fair but not good enough. Jon had uncovered enough that we could make out what appeared to be blackened curves that resembled the shape of a person lying on their side, one arm stretched out over the head and two legs that might be open, scissor-like. There were no fine features or gradients of shade to offer more complete clues.

Jon jammed the figure, the whole of it jiggling, meaning it was one piece. I took a turn and probed at what looked like the foot end. Blue. Not blue like the water bottle labels but an aqua blue. It wasn't cloth. The color revealed a shape like maybe the profile of a sandal. It was only maybe three inches long and blended into the surrounding gray-black. I jammed the staff as close as I could without hitting what was blue, the end signaling a rubbery, maybe woody, feeling.

Jon took another turn and stopped, pulling the length of the probe out of the pit and tossing it to the ground. We both got off of our knees.

"You don't think it's him, do you?" I asked Jon.

"I do. Maybe," he hedged. "What do we say?"

I looked at Jon, his eyes intent on mine as we huffed spit into our masks, both of us now at full sweat in our packaging. "I brought up the possibility earlier but everyone pretty much dismissed it. To be honest, I only considered the possibility since it was the one place we didn't look."

Jon turned towards the back of the unit, sweeping his arm across the horizon, saying, "And did anyone look out there?"

Out over the landscape was mile upon uninterrupted mile of low brush interspersed with palm and low trees. I was pulled back by the nagging thought of how little boys are drawn to fire. Other children had been shooed away a couple of times from the fire pit but it wasn't generally an issue. Finally, I concluded to Jon, dejectedly saying, "He could be anywhere."

Without ever answering each other if we should say something, we decided it was best to stay quiet. What purpose would be served since no one knew who the family was or where he came from. We weren't even certain if his name was his true name or how he arrived. What we did know was he was gone. Vanished into thin air. It was better to imagine he was a carefree 8 year old boy who was resourceful enough to find his own way home without much trouble. Never mind that he was not medically cleared.

Jon and I went our separate ways after doffing. He was tired and probably sought out his cot. I wanted to shower, clean up and get some sleep before the trip back to Freetown for the Sunday flight out of Africa. Several of the team members who had been assigned to field work wanted to make one last round before the trip home, giving me time to get some sleep and enjoy the rest of the day without feeling like I should be in bed.

Morning round was a quick review of all the patients, possible discharges and previous day's deaths. The survival rate was now approaching 75% of patients admitted in the last two weeks, the kind of improvement that elicits fist pumps and smiles. Nevertheless, the backdrop was always those who didn't make it out and one visit to the cemetery down the road was display enough why there really was nothing to celebrate, no more than putting out a fire at a house that has burned to the ground is cause to celebrate. It was as if a permanent curtain of black bunting shrouded your thoughts. Enough. I'm going home.

▪▪▪

Ali's Boots

Down the front of the unit, cars and vans were lined up dropping off replacements for those of us shipping out. J Edgar was busy trying to follow soccer highlights on the radio, allowing me to avoid saying some sort of awkward goodbye. None of the other usual gang knew that some of us were leaving, so it was the usual 'good mornings' and 'Reeeck!' greetings.

Past the main gate, Ali was at his table taking temps and making sure all the arrivals and departures were misted and washing their hands. I lined up with everyone else for the same.

"Good morning, Ali," I said. "You know what day it is?"

"Saturday," he replied, scanning my temple at the same time and writing it down.

I leaned down and untied the steer hide work boots on my feet, slipped out of the pair and put on the running shoes I brought with me. Then I plopped the boots on Ali's table, ordering, "Try these on. If they don't fit, I'm giving them to Racin."

I was teasing him, but was worried that if they didn't fit it would be a waste to not give them to someone who would. Ali looked concerned. The few people in line behind me crowded in closer to get a look, as if it was some sort of Cinderella's slipper moment.

"Try 'em. If they fit they're yours," I cajoled.

Ali sat down in his chair and kicked off his work issued rubber knee-high boots. Everyone had pulled in closer, some offering opinions on whether Ali would fit or not. Ali grabbed the left boot and slipped into it with no problem and laced it up with ease..

"Stand up," I gestured. Then I leaned over and checked to see where his toe placed. "Hey, about right," I smiled up at him.

He put on the right boot, laced it and took a few steps, his whole head all teeth and grin.

"Well, that's it. They're yours, Ali. Bye," I said, waving.

Before I could turn to walk out, Ali stopped me to give his thanks for the boots. It obviously made his day. I wished him the best, imploring him to take care of himself and be careful.

Outside, my ride back to the compound waited and we headed out. A breakfast was set aside for me so I had a quick bite and took one last bucket bath. I had packed the day before to avoid any last minute rush, finding out that I had lost my own cell phone. No big deal since I was going to be given a burner phone as part of the 21-day quarantine follow up once we landed in the United States.

It was a quick four hours of sleep, enough to leave me feeling refreshed when Adam knocked on my door to wake me up for the trip back to Freetown. It was good to have the original group back together and share our thoughts as Ibrahim wound us down the highway through the various Ebola check points.

Freetown in the daylight is a mass of humanity tucked into boxes of tin and stick punctuated by the occasional residential estate walled off from the rest of the country. Trash everywhere, especially spent 250 ml bags of drinking water. The Major decided to stay behind for the whole of Saturday and Galleo would be staying at the government hospital until mid February to help. Dr. Peterson was put on a morning flight out and was in the air heading home to Colorado. Gwyn and Jeanine had connections in the country from previous visits, staying on to refresh old friendships and continue other aid work.

Sunday morning, we spent time at a private beach, the birthplace of Atlantic hurricanes that slide off the west coast of Africa to torment North America between June and November every year. The contrast of where four of us ate lunch and swam was juxtaposed in my mind with images of Ali in his prized boots, monitoring the comings and goings of staff back at Maforki. The candle on our table kept reminding me of the fire pit, both humorous and disturbing, a maybe not so mysterious conclusion to a missing person after Jon and I finished poking around in it.

Soon enough we boarded our boat for the ferry trip to Lungi Airport and caught the plane to Brussels and into Newark Liberty. In Newark, we were all separated from the rest of the travelers and ID'd as Ebola workers. Uncle Sam had a system of interviews in place by US Navy medical staff, information on how and where to report to our local health departments and the free burner phone with a direct number to the Centers for Disease Control. It was efficient and informative and, soon enough, we were waved through customs, finally branching off our separate ways to catch our individual flights. I'm not sure if I felt as if I was abandoned or was abandoning our group.

Back home for me, quarantine was uneventful. I was allowed to move freely about the state, reporting in twice a day via video conferencing to report my morning and evening temperature. Others in the group, who had returned to other states, were separated from family, stern restrictions placed on them regards going out in public. I had the luxury of being home with my wife to appreciate her company and comfort, proving the adage that absence does make the heart grow fonder.

As the Midwest winter screwed itself back into my bones, I slowly came to internalize the tragedy I had witnessed, grieving for the Isatus and Mariatus and relief for the Kargbos. Any nonchalance or ambivalence I had in me about life not being fair as an impermeable, unmovable state of affairs was utterly destroyed. 'Is' absolutely does not have to be 'will be'. Optimism and elbow grease will change the odds if a person can force themselves out of the routines that keep them in their learned comfort zones. It is complete nonsense we have control over our fates when so much depends on such simple chance as where we are born and having permission from others to even try to participate. If nothing else came of all the efforts, I can at least look back and know that Ali ended up with a decent pair of boots.

Epilogue

If the Ebola crisis had emerged in the US with similar numbers infected as in Sierra Leone, the US health system would have been paralyzed. The generally beneficial hyper attention hospitalized patients receive in the US that manifests itself in slavish devotion to testing, multiple daily exams, divvying up of a single patient amongst multiple specialists and hypercharting would likely continue as usual. The first excuse to resist refiguring the health delivery system in such a crisis would be stated as lawsuit prevention, when the reality is that health care professionals are just as inured in routine and resistant to change as any other profession. Certainly, some enterprising malpractice lawyers would find fault in such a crisis and seek to capitalize, citing as cause any response that was less than fully ideal as most patients currently enjoy.

The philosophical rub that spawns malpractice suits is the ideal outcome vs the realistic outcome. Even when the standard of care is met, it is the unachieved ideal that often motivates legal retaliation, not negligence. A serious epidemic would strain our system not by numbers of sick alone but by failure to reconfigure the normal paradigm of care.

One example to consider is what happened after Hurricane Katrina. Memorial Hospital of New Orleans was flooded and made an island unto itself, stranding staff and patients for nearly two weeks with limited electricity, no air conditioning in sweltering mid-90's, Southern heat and no way in or out of the hospital other than small boats and a dicey helipad. Normal responses to emergent or urgent medical developments were suspended in favor of comfort care, especially in the critical care units. Morphine and other narcotic painkillers and sedatives were given to certain patients who had been under treatment for weeks or months, even years, for painful, terminal conditions, their tolerance for such narcotics having increased dramatically over the course of time, necessitating eye popping large doses to achieve the same effect a virgin to narcotics would need to ameliorate pain. Further complicating matters was the presence of a private for-profit hospital within Memorial devoted to high critical patients, many on ventilators, whose lives were being prolonged as part of a for-profit business model even when no hope of recovery was possible. It was many of these patients who became the casualties of disaster triage, in no small part thanks to the utter chaos and lack of reliable communication with the home office or evacuation officials.

Louisiana Attorney General Charles Foti, Jr. ordered an investigation and arrests after being led to believe the narcotic doses administered in some cases were intentionally lethal, that the doctor and several nurses practiced a triage type of euthanasia. The prosecutor first allowed himself not to be swayed by opposing medical opinion but instead relied on 5 physicians who had a stunningly brittle grasp of how narcotics work, especially in those who have been treated with opiates over long periods.

They say hindsight is 20-20, but even in the Memorial disaster, no clear answers appear. The doctors and nurses of Memorial were forced to triage the patients and ration care. There are nine recognized triage systems in healthcare. In a finger pointing culture like ours, it's easy to argue the other eight triage systems are superior in order to bludgeon the ninth choice. Hospitals usually pick one and train to that system. However, the fire departments and ambulance services may well have another and emergency disaster response of local or state government may still have another. Even if fortune had everyone using the same system, there still would have been arguable calls made on who received life-preserving care and who received comfort measures. Normally, the thinking is the sickest and most vulnerable get the first attention but in a disaster scenario, is that wise to withhold care from less sick patients more likely to survive? When you're in the disaster, you no longer have the luxury of relaxed reflection with no consequences as ideas are mulled over. Studies of personnel charged with triage have shown that those trained in the same system still have very widely different assessments. What may be a great system for one disaster may well be a lousy system for another.

In my own nursing experience with narcotics, I had more than a couple of patients who could tolerate very high doses that would have killed 'normal' patients. One such case was a teenage African-American who suffered from sickle cell anemia, a very painful blood condition. Her tolerance for morphine over one year increased to a level where we could push by IV 100 mg per dose as often as every two hours. A patient coming into the ER with a broken leg after falling off a ladder would likely receive 2-5mg IV initially and then about 2-4 mg IV every hour.

The physicians advising the New Orleans prosecuting attorneys probably saw doses charted by the storm stranded Memorial staff that were out of the range of what 'normal' patients would receive, but had no grasp of the doses many long term sufferers of chronic pain needed to achieve adequate control. With terrible consulted medical advice as a guide, the Louisiana AG set off on a crusade to prosecute, taking a natural disaster of immense scale that forced health care professionals to improvise, and then used that evidence of improvisation forced by unimaginable natural circumstances to define criminal acts by way of comparison with best practices during routine times. Many physicians who learned of individual patient circumstances lined up against the State of Louisiana. In testimony and letters, solicited and unsolicited, to officers of the court, they tried in vain to explain the nuances of narcotic administration and that it is not a one size fits all deal. The AG didn't care. The same AG had to be brow beaten into even considering investigating New Orleans police officers involved in highly questionable police on civilian shooting deaths. Eventually, after several years of dragging innocents around by the neck, a grand jury that did not hear from one single medical expert, a very intentional arrangement by the AG, told the AG to more or less go jump off a levee.

With such incidents as a backdrop in the back of hospitals' minds, no doubt they'd attempt to overcompensate in trying to protect themselves by adhering to an overly optimistic standard of care. Ebola patients would turn hospitals upside down. The risk of contagion alone requires extraordinary measures and resources to achieve safe isolation. Even with more routine bugs like MRSA (methycillin resistant staph aureus) and clostridium difficile, both potentially fatal, the US system of hospital infection control has failed miserably. It was and still is not at all uncommon for a hospital floor nurse to be assigned 5 to 6 patients per shift and have one of those patients be infected with MRSA or C difficile. That nurse must gown, mask and glove to administer patient care to such patients and be cognizant of how they dispose of their protective gear and how they wash. However, that nurse is still in the same scrubs and, rest assured, they didn't wash their face. As people we touch ourselves all over to scratch and itch or whatever, infecting our hands and then touching computer keyboards and other tools of work as we move on to the remaining patients of the assignment. It is absurd that hospitals continue this practice of mixing infected, contagious patients with uninfected patients and house them in rooms next to one another. In some cases, a contagious patient is assigned the same room with a non contagious patient when bed space is at a premium. This practice continues, though it is definitely on its way out, but not yet to the extent where contagious patients get their own part of the hospital building.

I mention Memorial Hospital and Hurricane Katrina to illustrate how in a disaster everything changes. Remember, that was one hospital in one city in one event of two weeks where every instrument of a government that is the most powerful and most organized on the face of this earth responded. When that government failed, it turned the power of the legal system on those caught in the maw of a natural disaster, attempting to extract a pound of flesh from the actors at Memorial in a display of power that risked zero to themselves. None of this is different than the politicians who beller about zero tolerance and getting tough on crime while excusing themselves from any accountability. In other words, cowards wearing ties who believe their public impression is all that matters. Many of these same cowards were given government escort and protection to achieve safe place as the storm lashed the city they swore to protect, having fled instead then returned to act out self righteously by targeting those who made the mistake of risking their own health and safety. Coward is a strong word but what other word can describe such people?

How did the general population of the United States respond to the news of an Ebola case in Texas? Total freak out. One single case. Thomas R Duncan, a Liberian national who visited relatives in Dallas, arrived infected and ended up in the Dallas Presbyterian emergency room complaining of a fever. He was sent home with the treating ER doc chalking it up to the flu. Only later was it learned that Duncan's port of exit was Liberia, a country in the thick of the Ebola crisis. He returned to the same ER and a correct diagnosis made but the previous couple of days he had spent with family, contagious. News media covered the whole debacle heavily but the fault was not in the reporting, but in the general public response.

Public response was outrage and panic. Many media outlets went to great pains to emphasize the real world odds of becoming Ebola infected but that didn't matter. Why? Honestly, my guess is that Americans enjoy such a relatively safe quality of life that they find it exciting to imagine they are on the cusp of some great disaster. A sense of impending doom was reinforced by certain politicians and the undercurrent was xenophobic, extending to accusations that Ebola infected Muslim terrorists were going to cross the US southern border with intentions to infect the American public. It certainly does not help when various media figures promulgate such utter idiotic nonsense in pursuit of ratings.

Further complicating matters was that one of the nurses caring for Mr. Duncan became infected. Soon enough we learned that the training she and her coworkers received was less than stellar and that those charged with Mr. Duncan's care had exposed skin. The CDC itself in the meantime issued advice and guidance from a distance, creating a perception of not being totally committed. Eventually, the CDC did become more forceful and hands on but had in the meantime squandered a fair amount of good faith.

When the CDC came on board to condemn the hysteria and issued hard and fast guidelines of how to identify a potential Ebola victim and how to treat them, hospitals put together plans of action, likely mostly to reassure the public they served they were 'doing something'. Ultimately, the real test was if anyone fitting the criteria of a potential Ebola victim showed up at the door. Thankfully, very few did, saving us all from the exercise of savage after the fact judgment that would waste time and effort on a real crisis.

When one nurse who served Ebola victims in West Africa returned home in November of 2014, perfectly healthy, New Jersey Governor Chris Christy imprisoned her in a tent in a hospital parking lot as part of her quarantine process. To the stupid, Governor Christy looked tough, though I'm quite sure he didn't lose a wink of sleep or miss connecting with whomever he wished at whatever time he wished. Many who backed the governor's stance cited 'you can never be too careful', but probably are the same types who will tell you with a straight face that wearing a helmet for riding motorcycle is silly, seatbelt laws are a constitutional violation and keeping a loaded firearm in the house is a reasonable safety measure.

Eventually the nurse was released from New Jersey to her home state of Maine. More political grandstanding occurred by Governor Todd Le Page who threatened involuntary forced seclusion of the nurse. There the nurse took a stand and had the unmitigated gall to go for a fall countryside bike ride. Again, politicians elected allegedly to protect Americans, decided it was great TV to pile on this particular American despite the fact that she was about as dangerous as a baby rabbit against a riding lawnmower. A judge heard the case and told the State of Maine to take a leap, finding the State of Maine's case to be all politics and no science.

With the aforementioned incidents, minor by any assessment, imagine 12,000 cases of Ebola in the United States. The American public would have had ample enough evidence to justify in their minds a panic of outrageous responses regardless of civil liberties. Our health system of detail and observance of strict protocol would become overwhelmed trying to treat the infected patients while simultaneously trying to reassure the public. At Dallas Presbyterian, an entire hospital floor was shut down for one patient. Now imagine an Ebola positive patient who took an airline ride, got in a taxi, rode the subway and stayed at a hotel. That would be a legitimate concern and contact tracing would need to be put into action, meaning every person the infected was in close proximity to would have to be identified and informed to report any signs or symptoms. It would consume several thousand man hours easily quarantining what could be literally hundreds of people showing no signs of illness just off one person's illness. The only sensible approach in a mass outbreak in order to prevent a health infrastructure meltdown would be to rely on strict public hygiene and self reporting.

Ebola is contagious and frighteningly fatal if not treated correctly, promptly. Yet the seasonal influenza takes upwards of 30,000 lives annually in the United States and about all we hear is some meager encouragement to get a flu shot. Of course, most of us have had the flu at one time or another and survived. However, part of the reason many of us caught the flu is that employer and school policies, while mouthing 'stay home and get well', still black mark employees and students for using sick days, coerce them to use vacation days or simply don't pay wages for the missed days. What happens is workers show up sick to take one for the team, needlessly infecting the well. Would an Ebola type crisis change American workforce thinking? To a degree but it would very likely take government intervention to protect employees from employer retaliation or other onerous sanctions. Employers might still ding employees with negative assessments for failing to show up for work, placing the burden completely on employees to make the call about their own employment record that they know will follow them.

In an odd sort of way, Sierra Leone was culturally more sympathetic to Ebola victims. Maybe it was the fact they were in the thick of it and the realization that it was dumb luck that stood between the sick and well. Also, Sierra Leone runs about a 70% unemployment rate, so the issue of work place transmission is significantly less of a problem. Of course, there are many stories of Ebola survivors not being allowed back into their communities for fear they would continue to be vectors. My take on the sympathy aspect is bolstered by how many families and friends of Ebola victims took great pains to care for their sick on their own and ensure a traditional burial, knowing they were at risk in comforting the ill and washing the bodies of the dead. The only rational solution to stemming the spread was to prevent such actions through organized intervention to stop such practices, deepening the national grief that so many victims were not traditionally funeraled.

Sierra Leone's history of civil unrest in the recent past contributed to the health care system being dysfunctional. Neighboring Liberia endured Charles Taylor's reign of terror but not before Taylor involved himself in Sierra Leone's civil war, committing atrocities of murder, rape and his army's signature maiming of chopping off the hands or arms of his opponents and his opponents supporters. Sierra Leone was pushed back to less than zero and today NGO's are attempting to help rebuild and train national medical personnel with the goal being to leave behind a self sustaining system that can mount vaccination programs, deliver reliable trauma care and make meaningful preventive health programs widely accessible. The success such an endeavor will need to overcome the distrust donor nations harbor towards Third World African countries and how pledged funds are handled.

It is fair to say that palms are greased, but the mistake that donor nations too often make is to accuse recipient nations of graft and corruption, meantime simultaneously steering such monies towards their own favored friends and supporters, often times who are not the best people for the job. I'll be the first to tell you that my eyes glaze over in putting forth a solution, but that is a poor excuse to stand back and do nothing. Accountability does matter; there needs to be a level of trust that the indigenous people are able to identify and prioritize their own needs best.

Where there is a lack of structure to inform, direct, inspire confidence and hope, facilitate personal and social growth, that is where there is a vacuum. Where there is a vacuum, something will move in to fill the void. Liberia and Sierra Leone saw that on the political level several decades ago, and in moved the warlords. More recently, the economic vacuum is being filled by foreign corporations and governments who are extracting a considerable amount of natural resources, the bulk of profits and royalties leaving the country, literally carried to the borders on the backs of citizens who endure subsistence challenged wages, physical abuse and wage theft. More than a few are children, forced against their will to haul product up out of the muck of mines.

Weak government unable to support a public health care system or lack of a strong, broad consumer class to support a vigorous free market health system, created yet another identifiable vacuum, which in this case was filled by Ebola. Ebola was not a new arrival by any stretch. High infant mortality, pedestrian bacterial infections such as cholera or insect borne parasitic diseases like malaria, hold their own, no true threat of eradication or meaningful control in the near future. Even the most simple and affordable methods of disease control, like soap and water, are subsumed by the need for relief from persistent and crushing poverty. On my river trip with Baker, I noticed some fishing nets rolled up off the sides of boats and thought it interesting they were such a fine mesh. Later, I figured out that these were mosquito nets handed out as part of a malaria prevention program. The locals found the nets to be good for fishing. There was no real choice. Either use the net to eat for certain today, or take a calculated risk when you sleep.

As I write these last words, Sierra Leone is still counting new Ebola cases, though as of October 31, 2015 they are about one a week and counting down through the 42 days of no new Ebola cases to be able to declare themselves Ebola clear. Liberia achieved that status early in the summer of 2015. Neighboring Guinea continues to smolder with about 1-2 cases per week, the rural areas presenting access issues for trained workers to get in and bolster eradication efforts.

Per the World Health Organization, a total, 28,109 cases world wide of Ebola as of the end of August, 2015. All, except for 34, occurred in the three West African countries of Sierra Leone, Guinea and Liberia. Sierra Leone reports the most cases at 13,609 with 3,953 deaths, followed by Liberia at 10,672 cases and 4,808 deaths and then Guinea at 3,792 cases of which 2,529 were fatal. (http://apps.who.int/ebola/ebola-situation-reports) The mortality rate of Guinea is clearly the worst of the three while Sierra Leone shows a better than 7 of 10 chance of survival. Tragically, part of Sierra Leone's reason for better survival rates is the Ebola crisis was so much larger over a longer period of time, giving responders a chance to refine treatment and prevention approaches, eventually having a working system in place for emergent cases as the outbreak wore on.

How the world responded to the Ebola outbreak is a mix of disconcerting and admirable. The disconcerting is that many people already present in West Africa to assist with economic and health system support bailed when the gravity of the situation became apparent. The number of those who left versus those who stayed behind is fuzzy, no organization exactly bragging publicly how many of their workers and volunteers exited. In the face of large unknowns and a larger known, i.e. a very high risk of death, the members of aid organizations faced a stark choice to preserve their own lives or risk them. For me to stand in judgment of those who left would be tantamount to judge a person who refused to rush into a burning building to try to save someone's life. Those kinds of judgments serve no purpose other than self aggrandizement of the person doing the judging, risking nothing.

The admirable aspects of the response came from organizations such as Doctors Without Borders that were present in the beginning, keeping what infrastructure they had in place as best they could, sticking with it throughout the worst. Other organizations that had no presence in West Africa prior to Ebola, ramped up quickly to recruit volunteers and workers to get into the thick of it, taking a two pronged approach of staffing Ebola Treatment Units for the immediate crisis and providing human and financial capital to woefully lacking clinics and hospitals in hopes of creating long term sustainability.

Governments as diverse as Cuba, United States and European nations responded with money, experts and people on the scene. For anyone who believes the world would be a better place without the United Nations, I'd show them the human infrastructure of the World Health Organization and how its presence facilitated the flow of vital information and acquisition of materials. The tendency to believe something is useless because we are not personally aware of what good it does us is often times an indicator of blunt ignorance we're not able to correct unless someone actively demonstrates the value.

The individuals who risked their own health? I peg them as rational and pragmatic arcing towards optimistic. Risk can be managed. If you asked them about being brave or heroic, they'd shake their heads at the absurdity of such a designation and point out that everyone else is too fearful. Those who responded were rewarded well, i.e. they had their curiosity satisfied and the need fulfilled to be of some help. They don't have to wonder what it was like, the same as Neil Armstrong one day no longer had to wonder what it's like to walk on the moon.

The joke around the compound always was, "How hard can it be?" the undercurrent of which is that our ignorance of what it truly takes to get some things done is what allows us to go forward. If we knew exactly what we were getting into, there's much we'd probably avoid.

In a sense, the Ebola crisis was approached like we in the United States approach terrorism--put the resources overseas so it doesn't land on our shores. Many politicians were convinced to release funding precisely to prevent further spread of the virus outside of West Africa, and that of course is perfectly fine. However, there was the usual grumbling from the typical quarters how it was a waste to use US tax dollars to ease another country's peoples' suffering, claiming the same funds should be spent back in the US to lock down the borders. Senator David Vitter (R)-LA was one such lawmaker who was unable to make the intellectual transfer of similarity between the fight against terrorism and disease. In fairness to the Senator, he had plenty of support in his shortsighted approach, but the 2014 lame duck Congress approved just over 6 billion, a victory of the pragmatic over ideology.

What does the future look like for Ebola? Anyone who claims with any certainty that they know needs to be dismissed as a crank. What we know is that as of the autumn of 2015, Ebola continues to smolder with a case here, a case there. The populace of West Africa is much more aware of the signs and symptoms and how to practice care and hygiene that reduces risk. However, Africa's history of frequent civil unrest poses the most ominous threat which could undermine essential defensive social infrastructure against another outbreak. Further clouding of what may or may not happen comes from recent research that concludes we aren't at all sure what the typical reservoirs are for the Ebola virus. Researchers thought certain species of fruit bat were Ebola reservoirs but now many are thinking that the level of antibodies identified aren't convincing enough to claim they are a regular host of the disease, that such levels merely indicate exposure at one time or another.

If you wonder why such knowledge matters, the best analogy I can make is John Snow's discovery during the 1854 Soho district of London cholera outbreak and how his work created the idea of focus of infection, i.e. where an outbreak originates. Snow found that a singular public pump was the culprit and when the pump was shut down, the outbreak subsided. A more relevant illustration many of us are familiar with is the seasonal flu bug and schools, that near perfect mix of lots of kids with questionable hygiene in close proximity, spreading out daily like spokes on a wheel to their families. Knowing where something comes from and how it travels goes a long ways in being able successfully to respond.

There is no perfect system. Our human fallibility of competing ideologies and agnosis of so much leaves us groping in the dark. While being able to predict the future is hit and miss, we do understand how we can respond to crisis, that having certain systems and resources in place at the ready can be of great help. It takes a certain amount of discipline to allocate resources today to be set aside for an unknown future event. Moreover, it takes wealth beyond what is needed for today's immediate needs. Thankfully, there are people who do this for all of us quite well such as certain world armies, World Health Organization, Red Cross and the Mormon Church disaster response network amongst many, many others. Every day that passes where the equipment gathers dust is a good day it doesn't have to be deployed. However, count on the fact that there will be a 'some day' again, about the only thing we can say with any certainty regards humanity's history. The impression left on me is that the need for universal health care is the only moral and affordable alternative. All in so we're all in.

There is still a very strange concept lingering in the United States that a person must earn the right to get medical care. How in the hell do you earn the right to medical care? The only criteria in that case is you earn the right to health care as long as you can shovel money into the system. After a person runs out of money, then they no longer have an earned right to health care? That'd be like Jesus healing the blind only after payment arrangements are made upfront. Yet many are convinced that for profit medicine is the way to go, though I'm not sure who wins the arguments in such boardrooms. Is it the patient with six figure medical needs who has a four-figure checking account or the duty to shareholders? If you'd like a peek at how such works out, look up Valeant Pharmaceuticals or Turing Pharmaceuticals CEO Martin Shkreli, both pathetic excuses of a collection of human beings that have monopolized certain drugs in order to gouge desperately ill patients.

How hard can it be to create systems where we all have access, a fair shot? If we continue to measure each other's worth in the size of wallets, fewer and fewer of us will be able to access the system as it continues to outpace inflation. The first real step to a solution is to dismiss the ideologues for the fools they are and force a public admission of values. The belief that a shareholder is more important than a patient is a value judgment, albeit a very twisted, naïve value that diminishes even the believer's own worth. Make opponents of universal global health care explain how profit is a moral triumph over the Good Samaritan. It should be an interesting explanation. Then ask yourself whom you want in charge during an Ebola type crisis.

Author's Note

The people and events in this book are at times composites of several people or events. All the events of which I have written are my own personal recollections, though in several instances I have used third party reports from my coworkers as my own. The names of the persons I worked with and the patients we served have been changed. The names of the people contained in the epilogue are true and accurate and my reporting of the events surrounding them have all been garnered from numerous newspaper and news program reports.

My special thanks to United States Agency for International Development and all the people throughout North America and Europe who performed admirably to achieve a response to the Ebola crisis. There is a book in of itself how that task was completed. My coworkers were inspiring and of great comfort. The Sierra Leonean nationals were equally supportive and wonderful. It is thanks to them that expatriates of all nationalities were able to work as well as we did. I carry each and every person in my heart every day.

November 2015

Cerebral Issue Press
New York, New York
10101

ABOUT THE AUTHOR

Richard Mertens is a Registered Nurse who lives a non-descript life in a non-descript part of the Midwest where he pines for the forests, lakes, mountains and oceans. In the meanwhile, he is cared for by his wife and pets who remind him that living in a sea of corn is tolerable when you're surrounded with friends.

Contact Information:

CerebralIssuePress@outlook.com

Subject line: Author Mertens